The 4-Day Wonder Diet

The 4-Day Wonder Diet

LOSE 10 POUNDS IN 4 DAYS

Margaret Danbrot

BANTAM BOOKS
TORONTO · NEW YORK · LONDON · SYDNEY · AUCKLAND

THE 4 DAY WONDER DIET

A Bantam Book/March 1986

ISBN 0-553-17191-7

Bantam Books are published by Bantam Books, Inc. Its
trademark, consisting of the words "Bantam Books" and
the portrayal of a rooster, is Registered in U.S. Patent and
Trademark Office and in other countries. Marca Regis-
trada. Bantam Books, Inc., 666 Fifth Avenue, New York,
New York 10103.

Printed and bound in Great Britain by
Cox & Wyman Ltd., Reading

With love, to Lisa and Bruce

CONTENTS

The 4-Day Wonder Diet

ONE

The 4-Day Wonder Diet: The Great New "Underground" Diet Revealed!

"THE DIET." For the last couple of years, that's how it has been referred to among the savvy and select group of women who used it time and again to take off weight fast. They also called it "great," "terrific," "a lifesaver," "the fastest diet in the West."

And though it didn't have a real name, it didn't need one. The flight attendants and retailing executives, the copywriters and the editors and bank officers who tried it and swore by it, all knew what you meant when you talked about "the diet."

Where the diet came from is a mystery. No one even knows the identity of the mastermind who first put it together. But everyone who tried it discovered the only really important thing they wanted to know about the diet...it works!

So, for years, women employed by the airlines and in editorial and retailing and editorial offices and banks photocopied the diet on plain paper and circulated it among their friends and co-workers...who in turn photocopied it for *their* friends and co-workers. In time, it became a sort of underground phenomenon. And like so many other underground phenomena—the excellent but unpublicized book or movie, the extraordinary little out-of-the-way restaurant, for example—this one attracted growing numbers of devoted fans via word of mouth ... because it works!

Naturally, a diet this good couldn't stay buried forever. And here it is: the Four-Day Wonder Diet.

Why is the Four-Day Wonder Diet so fabulous?

Because with this incredible no-nonsense, easy-to-stick-to diet, your minor weight problem will vanish in less than a week.

You can be five, seven, even ten pounds thinner in a short four days. Think of it!

When nothing in the closet fits the way it did when you bought it ... when shirts and pants begin to strain across the rear, and tummy bulge spoils your side-view silhouette, when the fabric of your blouse gapes open between the buttonholes ... and you have to suck in and tug hard to get your zippers to zip and your waistband ends to meet ... this is the diet that will help you and your clothes look chic again. And it will take only days, not weeks!

When a last-minute invitation to weekend at the beach means you just must get into bathing-suit shape, fast, you can start this diet on Tuesday and be bikini sleek by the time you hit the sand on Saturday morning!

When a series of high-pressure, high-cal business lunches begins to show, you can get rid of the evidence with the Four-Day Wonder Diet over a long weekend!

When splurging during the holidays or on vacation results in a five-pound gain, the Four-Day Wonder Diet can turn it into a net loss before anyone but you even notices!

When you're simply *feeling* fat and unattractive—whether you actually *look* it or not—the Four-Day Wonder Diet will restore your mood and your self-image to fit and fantastic practically overnight!

When, after weeks of exquisite torture and endless nervous nibbling to ease the tension, you finally manage to conquer the cigarette habit, only to find yourself—alas—a few pounds heavier than when you took your last puff, try the Four-Day Wonder Diet. Within a few days you'll be your old, slim self again, and healthier than ever.

When you want a shot of pure, unadulterated motivation to get you off to a flying start on a long-term weight loss program, you can use the Four-Day Wonder Diet as a kind of "pre-diet" diet. With it, you'll lose up to ten pounds in less than a week, and in the process feel so good about yourself that heightened self-confidence will keep you going when you switch gears into a slower-paced diet for the long haul.

However, if like so many of the women who've been using the Four-Day Wonder Diet all along, your weight problem is a relatively small one—say, five or ten pounds—you may *never* need another diet. Use the Four-Day Wonder Diet once, to bring the problem under control. After that, eat anything you want, within reasonable limits. Splurge occasionally on the foods you love best, but try to eat sensibly and weigh yourself regularly. Then, if you begin to put on unwanted pounds again, simply shift back on the Four-Day Wonder Diet and the weight will practically melt away. In less than a week you'll be in great shape again.

Some women think of the Four-Day Wonder Diet as a marvelous new kind of "figure insurance." With this diet on hand, they know there's no reason why a small weight problem should ever balloon into a big one. They know they never have to worry about getting fat again. It can be the same for you.

WHAT THIS DIET IS...AND ISN'T

If you are of a skeptical turn of mind, the Four-Day Wonder Diet might sound almost too good to be true. Quite possibly you are wondering just about now whether there are any "catches" or gimmicks involved. The truth is, there are none.

The Four-Day Wonder Diet is based on wholesome, good-tasting food that is readily available. You can buy everything you need for the diet at any supermarket or corner grocery store.

You won't have to go out of your way to shop for hard-to-find exotica. No out-of-season tropical fruits, or vegetables with strange-sounding names.

You won't have to accustom yourself to peculiar, unfamiliar flavors, or force down unpalatable substances such as bran or spirulena.

You won't have to weigh or measure anything. On the Four-Day Wonder Diet, exact portion sizes are relatively unimportant. In fact, you can have as much as you like of some of the foods on the diet.

You won't have to count a single calorie, either, or do any tricky calculations with regard to making "exchanges" or substituting one food for another. There are no menus to plan, no alternative foods to consider, no choices to make. Everything is figured out for you in advance, so there's no guesswork on your part.

You *will* have to follow the Four-Day Wonder Diet to the letter. You must eat *only* the foods specified on the diet, and you must eat *all* of them. It's important not to skip any of the foods listed and except in special circumstances you must not replace them with other foods.

And you must eat them in the proper sequence. As

you will discover when you see the diet itself in the next chapter, breakfast is always the same. However, lunch and dinner are different on each of the four days. The sequence is an essential factor in the effectiveness of the diet. It's important that you adhere to that sequence exactly, eating *only* the foods listed for Day One on the first day, only the foods listed for Day Two on the second day, and so on, ending with the foods listed for Day Four on the fourth day. The success of the Four-Day Wonder Diet depends on it. You won't get the same marvelous results if you deviate from the sequence.

This is a diet that leaves nothing to chance. There's no margin for error. You can't possibly make a mistake in judgment as to whether a particular food is "allowed" or not. You won't ever have to wonder whether it's okay to substitute certain foods for others. The rules and regulations are all set down for you in black and white. If it's not specified on the Four-Day Wonder Diet, you don't eat it. If it's part of the diet, you *must* eat it.

Strict? You bet! But interestingly enough, it is this very strictness that accounts in large measure for the enormous success and appeal of the Four-Day Wonder Diet. You may be surprised to discover, like many Four-Day Wonder dieters before you, that never having to make food decisions simplifies the weight loss process. And that knowing in advance exactly what to eat and when makes losing pounds easier, not more difficult. This is often the case even for strong-willed types who ordinarily balk at being told what to do.

Having too many choices, it's been said, has been the downfall of many a dieter. But it's never a problem on the Four-Day Wonder Diet.

WHY THEY LOVE THE 4-DAY WONDER DIET

Anyone who's willing to follow the Four-Day Wonder Diet *to the letter* will be thrilled with the results. But for certain *kinds* of diet personalities—especially those who've had problems starting, and *staying,* on a diet in the past—the success of the Four-Day Wonder Diet has been nothing short of extraordinary. Maybe you'll recognize something of yourself in one of the following profiles.

The Sensuous Woman

She's attractive, with a healthy concern for her appearance, but she's much too easy-going and relaxed to be obsessed with her looks. Even so, she's fashion-conscious, mad about beautiful clothes in luscious fabrics, and looks smashing in up-to-the-minute styles.

She knows the rules of proper nutrition by heart and honestly tries to live by them. In fact, she's good about food much of the time and weighs approximately what she ought to, give or take a few pounds. But she *is* a bit of a hedonist. Her enthusiasm for life, and love, and all the sensual pleasures is practically boundless. She especially delights in the aromas, the textures, the tastes of good food, and sometimes she overindulges.

When the needle on the bathroom scale begins to edge upward, she naturally thinks about going on a diet. But as long as the problem remains a small one, her motivation stays low, and she may put it off. As a lover of the finer things, food included, she dreads the idea of denying herself. And as for mustering the will power and maintaining the discipline necessary to lose a few pounds slowly, over a period of weeks, on an ordinary diet...well, it makes her miserable just to think about it!

Whoever thought up the Four-Day Wonder Diet must have had the Sensuous Woman in mind. Unwanted pounds practically vanish overnight, and the whole weight loss process is over and done with almost before the dieter has a chance to miss the joys of eating!

Ms. Thirty-five Plus

She's loaded with energy, a real doer, and because she has always been so active, she has felt free to eat just as she pleased. Usually, that meant packing away three square meals a day, and nibbling on anything that interested her in between. Less fortunate friends marveled at her seeming ability to consume as much as she liked of whatever she liked, without any visible consequences.

What her friends didn't realize was that she *did* sometimes put on extra pounds. However, when her scale registered a small gain, she would simply cut back. Two or three days of "watching it"—eliminating snacks and sweets—was all it took to get her weight down.

Not anymore. Now that she is approaching forty, unwanted pounds pile on more quickly, and she is finding that her old technique of cutting out snacks and sweets doesn't work as well as it once did. She has discovered that not only must she eliminate snacks, but she must also eat smaller portions of everything else to get her weight down where she wants it, and keep it there. Her days of eating everything and anything are over.

She read someplace that upon approaching one's forties there is a natural and predictable slowing of the metabolism, and she realizes that's what is happening to her. She knows it's time to adjust her eating habits accordingly, and as soon as she can lose a few pounds, that is exactly what she plans to do. But first she has to lose that weight!

The Four-Day Wonder Diet is perfect for her. With it, excess pounds are blitzed away in less than a week. Going on the diet is almost as easy as "watching it" used to be. And if a few unwanted pounds creep back on, the Four-Day Wonder Diet will blitz them off again.

The Either/Or Eater

Like the Sensuous Woman, the Either/Or Eater is attractive and fashion-conscious. She loves being thin, the thinner the better. She might even be a teensy bit neurotic about her weight. She's positively phobic about fat. Gaining a few pounds can throw her into an emotional tailspin.

For her it's either famine or feast. She's aware of every bite she takes. Unfortunately, feelings of rejection or disappointment trigger in her an overwhelming urge to splurge on food. Often, she experiences a wild craving for sweets just before a period.

Binging, however, neither elevates her mood nor satisfies her cravings. Instead of pulling her up out of the dumps, the guilt and anxiety she feels about overeating— and perhaps gaining weight—tend to push her down even further. It can become a vicious cycle: she overeats when she feels unhappy; then the prospect of gaining weight makes her feel even more unhappy, which leads in turn to more overeating.

To break the cycle, the Either/Or Eater often finds that a strict, no-nonsense food regimen is helpful. And if that regimen will also quickly undo any damage done by a few days of binging, so much the better. The Four-Day Wonder Diet does just that. Pounds are gone within days, not weeks or months. For the Either/Or Eater, the Four-Day Wonder Diet is a marvelous tool that can put her back in control of her eating.

The Either/Or Eater really should try to get a grip on herself and develop a healthier outlook and more reasonable eating habits. (In extreme cases, professional intervention may be a good idea.) In the meantime, however, the Four-Day Wonder Diet can help her manage wild binging behavior and get back on a firmer food footing.

The Disappointed Dieter

She's smart, sensitive and savvy...and yet it seems that she's spent her entire adult life searching for the perfect diet. She's tried them all. Every so often a friend will recommend a new one, one that has worked wonders and resulted in an impressive number of pounds lost. But when the Disappointed Dieter tries it, she's...well, disappointed.

She starts each new diet with high hopes and high motivation. But, often by the end of the first week, and always by the end of the second, she's in despair. After two whole weeks of being good, of facing down temptation, of feeling hungry and deprived, she finds that she has lost only four or five pounds. The disappointment undermines her will to continue, and so she gives up.

A problem with many of the good, nutritionally sound reducing diets—the kind that have led to so much discouragement for the Disappointed Dieter—is that though they're safe and effective over the long run, they're also very *slow.* It can be weeks before there's a significant payoff in terms of pounds lost. Some people can wait it out, but not the Disappointed Dieter.

She needs extra help. The Four-Day Wonder Diet isn't meant for long-term weight loss, but it will reward her with an immediate, significant payoff. Momentum, plus the thrill of losing up to ten pounds in less than a week, can carry the Disappointed Dieter through the next few weeks of ordinary, safe, slow dieting. Better yet, when weight loss slows to a halt on her ordinary diet, she can switch back to the Four-Day Wonder Diet to speed things up again.

THE 4-DAY WONDER DIET: WHAT'S IN IT FOR YOU?

On the Four-Day Wonder Diet, you'll lose more than you ever thought possible in less than a week. Believe it or not, some people who've tried both say they've lost more pounds on the Four-Day Wonder Diet than they have on a fruit-juice and clear soup fast!

Now, what about you? How many pounds can you, personally, expect to lose on the Four-Day Wonder Diet?

It's impossible to make accurate, to-the-pound predictions. Too many different factors influence the amount of weight any individual dieter will lose. However, based on the following considerations, you should be able to make a pretty good "guesstimate."

Physical activity. As a general rule, the more active you are, the more weight you will lose on this—or any—reducing diet. (Nevertheless, be assured that the Four-Day Wonder Diet will work wonders for you, even if you are a sedentary type.)

It is best not to begin any new and strenuous exercise program while you are on a strict diet such as the Four-Day Wonder Diet. But with that caveat in mind, if you are in good health, you should be able to take advantage of the extra calorie-burning potential of *gentle* exercise. Boosting your activity level even slightly can result in greater weight loss. And who knows? You may enjoy your newly initiated exercise program so much that you'll be inspired to keep up the good work and make it a part of your daily routine after you've completed the diet. In

Chapter Eleven, you will find suggestions for starting and maintaining a fitness program, as well as special exercises for shaping and toning problem areas.

If you've already acquired the habit of regular, vigorous exercise, there's no reason why you shouldn't continue at your present high activity level throughout the Four-Day Wonder Diet.

Age is another factor that will influence the amount of weight you can expect to lose on a diet. All else being equal, women and men under the age of forty will lose more on the Four-Day Wonder Diet than those over forty. This is because of the gradual and inevitable metabolic slowdown that ordinarily begins during the late thirties. As your metabolism slows, your body requires fewer and fewer calories to maintain your weight. In fact, the number of calories you need to eat to keep your weight steady at age twenty might actually lead to a weight *gain* at forty!

Metabolic slowdown accounts, at least in part, for the increased difficulty in losing weight experienced by many people in their middle years. (A decrease in physical activity in those years often adds to the problem.)

But no matter what your age, you *will* lose pounds quickly and easily on the Four-Day Wonder Diet.

Your weight. The present state of your shape will also affect the amount of weight you will lose on the Four-Day Wonder Diet. The more you *need* to lose, the more you *will* lose. If you are only a few pounds overweight, you can expect to lose most or all of them by the time you've completed the diet. If you are twenty, thirty, or more pounds heavier than you should be, you might lose up to ten pounds in four days!

Your height and your body build. All else being equal, tall, large-boned people will ordinarily lose more weight on the Four-Day Wonder Diet (or any diet) than short or small-boned types. But even petites, with bones as slender and fragile as a bird's, will lose more weight than they ever thought possible in less than a week of Four-Day Wonder dieting.

WHY 4 DAYS TO FABULOUS... AND NO MORE?

When the four days are up, it's time to go off the Four-Day Wonder Diet, no matter how well it has worked for you. On the fifth day, resume normal eating, or move on to a less drastic diet that will help you get down slowly and surely to the weight you want to be.

If you must lose a significant amount of weight, you need a safe, sensible eating plan that will help you shed one and a half to two pounds a week, week after week, month after month. You can get a head start with the Four-Day Wonder Diet, or you can use it at the end, when you've lost most of the weight you wanted to lose and would like to finish off the last few pounds in a hurry. You can even use the Four-Day Wonder Diet once or twice in the middle weeks of a diet, when you've hit a plateau and want to start losing quickly again. But you should not use the Four-Day Wonder Diet for more than four days at a time.

The diet is a strict one. That's why it works. It does not offer well-balanced, textbook-perfect nutrition. On the Four-Day Wonder Diet, two important food groups are eliminated completely, while at the same time you are allowed to eat as much as you like of some others. The balance of foods offered by the Four-Day Wonder Diet is ideal for speedy weight loss, but it's not recommended for use over the long run.

If your goal is to lose more than ten or fifteen pounds,

ask a doctor to recommend a reduced-calorie regimen that will help you take the weight off slowly and sensibly. Or go to a bookstore or library and pick out one of the many good weight loss "classics." Even if you do decide to choose a diet for yourself, however, it is still important to check with a physician to find out if there is any reason why that particular diet may not be a good choice for you.

DOCTOR'S PERMISSION, PLEASE

For the same reason, check with your doctor before starting the Four-Day Wonder Diet for the first time. There are very few medical conditions that would preclude your going on the diet, but get an okay first, just in case.

And don't be surprised if your doctor doesn't love this diet. As you will soon see for yourself, it's super-low in some nutrients, super-high in others. That's part of the magic. It's not meant to be a substitute for lifetime good nutrition. But as a terrific, almost-instant problem-solver, there has never been anything quite like it!

TWO

The 4-Day Wonder Diet: The Basic Diet

YES, you *can* lose up to ten pounds in less than a week on the Four-Day Wonder Diet. Which means that if your weight problem is a relatively small one, you may be able to solve it *completely* over a long weekend. And if weekend dieting is inconvenient? Start on Tuesday or Wednesday and be visibly sleeker and slimmer by the following weekend!

All it takes is the desire to get thinner in a hurry! That, and a willingness to commit yourself totally to the diet. Remember, the Four-Day Wonder Diet is *strict*. It's going to demand a lot from you. But in return you'll get what you've always wanted most from a diet: fast, sure results.

Your first glance at the Four-Day Wonder Diet might leave you feeling somewhat puzzled. "It doesn't look that much different from some of the other diets I've tried," was one woman's immediate reaction. Your initial impression of the diet might be similar to hers.

But then she took a second, closer look and realized that the Four-Day Wonder Diet is indeed different.

The most obvious difference: Certain foods that one

expects to find on almost every weight loss diet are missing from this one.

For example, though you will find eggs on the Four-Day Wonder Diet, you won't find any other dairy foods. No milk, not even skimmed milk. No cheese, not even the low-cal cottage, Farmer, and pot cheeses that are staples on most reducing diets. No yogurt. And no butter or margarine—not even a single pat to relieve the dryness of breakfast toast!

And that's no wonder, because there is no bread on the Four-Day Wonder Diet. Not even thin-sliced, low-cal diet bread. There's no melba toast, either. In fact, the diet includes *no* foods from the grain/cereal category. That means no corn or bran flakes. And of course, no pasta.

The two major food categories that are omitted from the Four-Day Wonder Diet—dairy products and grains and cereals—are rich in nutrients important to good health. Most diets that are meant to be followed for long periods, and are planned to result in a slow and steady weight loss of one and a half to two pounds a week, include at least one or two servings a day of dairy foods and grain/cereal products. But these two food groups have no place on a short-term diet that promises to blitz off pounds in a hurry, and for a very important reason: they do nothing to accelerate the weight loss process.

You can safely do without dairy products for a few days. There's nothing magic about them. Don't forget, some perfectly healthy people rarely, if ever, drink milk or eat cheese, either because of allergies, or in some cases, because of simple dislike.

As for cereals and grains, no one would suggest that it would be a good idea to eliminate these valuable foods from your diet for months or even weeks. But you can safely skip them during the Four-Day Wonder Diet.

Now that you know what you won't find on this super-speedy, strict, but easy-to-follow diet, let's focus on what you will find.

Breakfast on each of the four days is the same:

>½ grapefruit
>Black coffee or tea

Lunch and dinner on Day One are as follows:

LUNCH Broiled steak or hamburger
     Lettuce and tomato salad, no dressing
     1 apple

DINNER 2 hard-boiled eggs
     Green beans
     ½ grapefruit

For lunch and dinner on Day Two, you may have the following:

LUNCH 1 lamb chop
     Lettuce, no dressing
     6 ounces tomato juice

DINNER Squash and cauliflower, steamed or raw
     6 ounces green beans
     Unsweetened applesauce

On Day Three, have the following foods for lunch and dinner:

LUNCH Lettuce and celery salad, no dressing
     Broiled chicken
     1 apple

DINNER Hamburger patty
     Stewed tomatoes
     6 ounces prune juice

Finish up on Day Four with the following foods:

LUNCH   2 hard-boiled eggs
           6 ounces green beans
           6 ounces tomato juice

DINNER   Broiled steak or hamburger
           Lettuce and tomato salad, no dressing
           6 ounces unsweetened pineapple juice

And there you have it: four days of low-calorie, low-carbohydrate, high-protein eating that will streamline your shape in less than a week!

HOW AND WHY IT WORKS

As you already know, the Four-Day Wonder Diet has been a hot underground phenomenon for two or three years now. It has been touted by word of mouth, photocopied and passed from one thrilled, pounds-thinner dieter to the next. Even with diligent checking, it hasn't been possible to discover the identity of the person who first created the Four-Day Wonder Diet. Under the circumstances, we can't know for certain exactly why he or she arrived at the specific mix of foods called for on the diet, or the sequence in which they are to be eaten. But we *can* make some educated guesses.

The Vegetables

First of all, notice the emphasis on vegetables. Cauliflower, celery, green beans, lettuce and summer squash or zucchini . . . all are extremely low in calories:

Cauliflower	1 cup	28 calories
Celery	1 cup	20 calories
Green beans	1 cup	34 calories
Lettuce	1 cup	10 calories
Squash	1 cup	30 calories

These vegetables are *so* low in calories that when you eat them, your body expends almost as much energy (calories) just to pick them up on a fork, swallow and digest them as the vegetables themselves supply!

Consider this: a 120-pound woman at rest—either seated quietly or lying down—burns calories at the rate of approximately twenty per half hour. (The figure is not exact; it would vary somewhat from person to person, but twenty is above average.) Calorie expenditure for that same woman rises to approximately forty-five per half hour during the process of eating a meal! A quick look at the chart above tells us that none of the vegetables on the Four-Day Wonder Diet supplies more than thirty-four calories per cup. It's easy to see why eating these vegetables—even in large amounts—adds practically nothing in real terms to your daily calorie intake.

In a sense, these vegetables can be considered "neutral" foods, because they supply so few calories and the calories they do supply are almost immediately expended just in the process of eating!

Don't be afraid to fill up on these vegetables. They'll take up space in your stomach and contribute to feelings of fullness at mealtimes. They'll also provide you with the much-needed sensory satisfaction (lacking in so many diets) of chewing and swallowing. And all at a minimal cost in calories. In fact, your jaws will begin to tire long before you can consume enough of these low-cal vegetables to upset the balance of the diet.

Now let's consider the other elements that help zip off pounds on the Four-Day Wonder Diet.

The Protein Foods

The most important of these other elements are the protein foods: eggs and hamburger, steak, lamb chops, and chicken. None of these are strikingly low in calories:

Eggs	2 medium	150 calories
Hamburger	3 ounces	185–250 calories, depending on fat content
Steak	3 ounces	250–350 calories, depending on fat content
Lamb chop	1, 1 inch thick	250–350 calories, depending on fat content
Chicken, no skin, no bone	3 ounces	120 calories

If you take another quick look at the complete Four-Day Wonder Diet, you will see that except for breakfast, which is grapefruit and coffee or tea on all four days, and dinner on Day Two, which is a vegetarian meal, most of the calories you consume will be supplied by protein foods. Protein is the dominant element of the diet.

When a diet is structured so that most of the calories are supplied by protein foods, an interesting process comes into play. In greatly simplified terms, protein—especially the protein in "animal" foods such as meat and eggs—tends to stoke up the body's metabolism, quickening the rate at which food is converted into energy, and in particular revving up the process by which the body burns off its own fat!

This process is thought to account for the results of some of the most fascinating of all weight loss studies.

These studies seem to indicate that with a diet high in protein there is a greater reduction in body fat than with a diet supplying calories primarily in the form of carbohydrate foods (sugars, starches, and so on). And this appears to be the case even when the protein foods are themselves relatively high in fat!

This increase in fat burnoff and the resulting rapid weight loss has been a factor in the success of many high-protein diets. Apparently, it is also one of the reasons why pounds melt away so quickly on the Four-Day Wonder Diet!

If you look back once again at the complete Four-Day Wonder Diet, you will see that no quantities are given for the steak or hamburger at lunch on Day One, for the broiled chicken at lunch on Day Three, or for the steak or hamburger at dinner on Day Four. You can eat as much as you like! (Within reason, of course.) When your stomach registers a nice, satisfied feeling, it's time to stop. (Never mind if there are a few more morsels on your plate. Whether you are dieting or not, it's always a good idea to "listen" to your stomach, and to stop eating when it tells you you've had enough, even though your taste buds cry for more!)

Fruits and Juices

Fruits and fruit juices make up the remainder of the diet. (Yes, botanically speaking, the tomato *is* a fruit!) The ones you will enjoy on the Four-Day Wonder Diet are higher in calories than the vegetables, but not much:

Grapefruit	½ small	60 calories
Apple	1 small	75 calories
Applesauce (unsweetened)	½ cup	50 calories
Tomato juice	6 ounces	38 calories

Tomato	1 medium	20 calories
Stewed tomatoes	1 cup	50 calories
Prune juice	6 ounces	148 calories
Pineapple juice (unsweetened)	6 ounces	103 calories

What do these fruits and fruit juices contribute to the Four-Day Wonder Diet? Vitamins, for one thing, and vitamin C in particular. Since vitamin C is not stored in the body, it is important to have an adequate supply of it each day. The half grapefruit at breakfast each morning fulfills this requirement. Your daily C supply is further augmented by smaller amounts of the vitamin in the other fruits and juices.

In addition, by supplying small but significant amounts of carbohydrates, the fruits and fruit juices help to prevent the accumulation of ketones. Ketones are organic compounds produced in the body when there are insufficient carbohydrates present during fat metabolization. Much of the criticism that has been leveled at some of the popular all-protein, no-carbohydrate diets stems from a concern over ketone buildup, which can lead to unpleasant feelings of fatigue and even nausea or dizziness—symptoms that can be frightening, to say the least, when their cause is not known.

Fruits, along with the low-cal vegetables on the diet, provide bulk, also known as fiber or roughage, which helps prevent constipation—a big problem on many diets. The prune juice is there for good measure!

Finally, fruits and juices provide a nice taste and texture change of pace. Save your fruit or juice for the end of a meal, and think of it as dessert. (Admittedly, they're not in the same league as chocolate cake ... but then chocolate cake is the enemy as long as you need to lose weight.)

CALORIE COUNTDOWN

Earlier, you learned that you don't have to count even a single calorie on the Four-Day Wonder Diet. You'll lose pounds and inches faster than you ever thought possible, simply by eating the foods specified for each day of the diet. Nevertheless, since almost everyone is calorie-conscious these days—no doubt because so many diets *do* stress the number of calories that may be consumed—let's look at the Four-Day Wonder Diet in a calorie context.

You will notice that the chart on pages 23–24 gives three calorie grand totals for Day One, Day Three, and Day Four. That's because on each of those days you may eat as much as you like of steak or hamburger, or in the case of Day Three, chicken. In each case, the lowest grand total has been calculated on the assumption that you will eat *four ounces of meat or chicken*. The second-highest grand total is based on your eating *six ounces of meat or chicken*. And the highest grand total assumes that you will eat *eight ounces of meat or chicken!* That's half a pound—much more than most people eat even when they're not concerned about their weight.

In every case, calorie counts for vegetables are calculated on the assumption that you will eat at least a cup of each.

You will note that there is only one calorie grand total for Day Two. That's because the amount of meat you may eat that day is fixed at a single lamb chop.

As you can see, on the Four-Day Wonder Diet, the number of calories that you consume daily might total anywhere from 550 to 1,081, depending on the amount of meat or chicken you fill up on. If you have a whopping

DAY ONE

BREAKFAST	½ grapefruit	60				
LUNCH	4-ounce steak	333	6-ounce:	499	8-ounce:	666
	1 cup lettuce	10				
	1 tomato	20				
	1 apple	75				
DINNER	2 hard-boiled eggs	150				
	1 cup green beans	34				
	½ grapefruit	60				
TOTALS		742		908		1075

DAY TWO

BREAKFAST	½ grapefruit	60
LUNCH	1 lamb chop	250
	1 cup lettuce	10
	6 ounces tomato juice	38
DINNER	1 cup squash	30
	1 cup cauliflower	28
	1 cup green beans	34
	1 cup unsweetened applesauce	100
TOTAL		550

DAY THREE

BREAKFAST	½ grapefruit	60				
LUNCH	4 ounces broiled chicken	160	6 ounces:	240	8 ounces:	320
	1 cup lettuce	10				
	1 cup celery	20				
	1 apple	75				
DINNER	4 ounces hamburger	248				
	1 cup stewed tomatoes	50				
	6 ounces prune juice	148				
TOTALS		771		851		931

DAY FOUR

BREAKFAST	½ grapefruit	60				
LUNCH	2 hard-boiled eggs	150				
	1 cup green beans	34				
	6 ounces tomato juice	38				
DINNER	4-ounce steak	333	6-ounce:	499	8-ounce:	666
	1 cup lettuce	10				
	1 tomato	20				
	6 ounces pineapple juice	103				
TOTALS		748		914		1081

eight ounces of meat on Day Four, and eight full ounces of chicken on Day Three, your total calories for those days will average out to about 1,000. (The calorie count for Day Two is fixed at 550.) Of course, as the chart indicates, you might consume significantly *fewer* calories if you eat less meat and chicken. But even if your calorie average is up around 1,000, you can still expect to lose pounds and inches fast on the Four-Day Wonder Diet.

THE 4-DAY WONDER DIET
VERSUS
THOSE LONG-DISTANCE DIETS

Many of the popular diets that are generally considered to be safe to follow for weeks and even months at a time allow the dieter an average of between twelve hundred and fifteen hundred calories a day. On those diets, a steady weight loss of approximately one-and-a-half to two pounds a week is predicted. The difference between the calories that you are allowed on those diets and the number you will consume on the Four-Day Wonder Diet is small. Yet,

on the Four-Day Wonder Diet, you might lose in excess
of two pounds a *day,* as compared to the two pounds a
week promised by the long-distance diets! How can this
be?

The best way to explain it is to point out again that
on the Four-Day Wonder Diet, protein foods are dominant, and greater-than-normal amounts of protein tend
to shift the body's metabolism into "overdrive," speeding
up the rate at which fat is burned off.

Consider this: If you eat eight ounces of steak or hamburger on Day One of the Four-Day Wonder Diet, almost
seventy-six percent of your total calories that day will
come from protein food. Further, if you eat eight ounces
of steak on Day Four, protein foods will contribute sev-
enty-five percent of your total daily calories. Even on Day
Two, which features a vegetarian dinner, and Day Three,
forty-five and sixty-one percent of your calories, respec-
tively, will come from protein food. Thus, the Four-Day
Wonder Diet is designed to maximize the high rate of
"fat burnoff" that is the result of consuming greater
amounts of protein.

But—and this is important—it is not necessary to eat
half a pound of meat or chicken to benefit from the super
fat-burning potential of protein food. Even eating only
four ounces of meat or chicken will supply you with more
than enough protein to obtain the accelerated fat-burning
benefits that zap away pounds in a fraction of the time
it takes on an ordinary diet.

THE ALL-IMPORTANT STRICTNESS FACTOR

Earlier on, the strictness of the Four-Day Wonder Diet was emphasized. Now that you know so much more about the diet, you may be wondering why it is characterized as "strict." After all, on three out of four days you may have approximately one thousand calories, and the way you divvy up those calories is left pretty much to your own discretion. The amount of meat you consume on Days One, Three, and Four is flexible. So is the amount of vegetables at *any* of the lunches and dinners.

The Four-Day Wonder Diet is flexible, yes. But flexible within a strict framework. We haven't yet touched on the few simple but ironclad dos and don'ts that make this perhaps the easiest and certainly the most effective diet you'll ever follow. You'll see why it has been said that nothing important has been left to chance, and why it is impossible to make a mistake! And you'll see why it has been emphasized that the Four-Day Wonder Diet asks a lot of you as a dieter. By the time you finish your first round, you'll *know* it was worth every ounce of extra effort you put into it!

THREE

Eleven Rules That Make You a Winner at Losing

No MATTER how much you want to begin losing pounds and inches on the Four-Day Wonder Diet, don't even *think* about starting it before reading this chapter from beginning to end. The important dos and don'ts explained here, along with the suggestions included for enhancing sure and speedy weight loss, can make all the difference between dieting failure and fast, fabulous success.

Some of the rules that follow might seem arbitrary and unnecessarily strict at first glance. But as you will soon see, there are reasons—*good* reasons—for every single one of them.

Here they are for ready reference. Explanations follow.

1. Do not vary, substitute, or delete any of the foods listed on the Four-Day Wonder Diet.
2. Don't eat *anything* between meals.
3. Don't drink alcoholic beverages of any kind.
4. Drink plenty of water while you are on the diet.
5. Have as much black coffee or plain tea as you like,

but limit diet soda to two twelve-ounce bottles
per day.
6. Eat vegetables raw, steamed, or boiled.
7. Broil all meat and chicken.
8. Remove all traces of fat from meat and chicken
before you eat it.
9. Use only salt, pepper, or lemon juice to season
food.
10. Fill up, but don't overdo it!
11. Don't stay on the Four-Day Wonder Diet longer
than four days.

*1. Do not vary, substitute, or delete any of the foods listed on
the Four-Day Wonder Diet.*

Though all of the rules that follow are important, this
one may be the most important of all. If a certain food
is not specifically listed as part of the diet, don't eat it!
As for the foods that *are* listed, you *must* have at least
some of each. There are only two valid reasons for bending
this rule:

Allergies. Naturally, you should not eat any food listed
on the diet if it has resulted in an allergic reaction in the
past. If you *are* allergic to something on the diet, you
should replace it with a similar food of comparable caloric
content. For example, if eggs, a protein food, are a problem, you should replace the two eggs listed for dinner
on Day One and for lunch on Day Four with another
protein food, such as chicken, hamburger, or steak to
equal the caloric content of the eggs. If you cannot eat
grapefruit, substitute another fruit that is also high in
vitamin C and supplies a comparable number of calories.
The substitution information below will help you make
necessary adjustments.

Budget considerations. The steak and lamb chops on the

Four-Day Wonder Diet are delectable and provide variety, but there's no quarreling with the fact that they are also expensive. If you're experiencing a temporary cash flow problem and don't mind a lack of variety, there will be little harm done in replacing these two pricey items with more chicken or hamburger. You may have as much chicken or hamburger as you like as a substitute for steak at lunch on Day One, and at dinner on Day Four. However, calories *are* a consideration if you decide to substitute either for the lamb chop at lunch on Day Two; at that meal you may have only enough chicken or hamburger to equal the calorie content of the chop (about 250 calories). If you need help in making this adjustment, see the substitution material below.

Food substitutions. As you know, substitutions are to be avoided on the Four-Day Wonder Diet. However, when allergy or expense (in the case of steak and lamb chops) make it impossible for you to follow the diet exactly as written, it is permissible to replace the problem food with another food of the same type (i.e., vegetable, meat/egg, or fruit) that supplies approximately the same number of calories.

That word "approximately" is important here. Few foods are exactly equal in the number of calories they supply per ounce or per serving, and several of the substitutions listed below are somewhat higher or lower in calories than the foods they are meant to replace. The difference should not affect the amount of weight you will lose on the diet if you eat the replacement foods in the amounts specified.

Vegetable substitutions. With the exception of lettuce, you may replace any vegetable on the Four-Day Wonder Diet with an equal amount of any other vegetable on the diet. Or you may replace any vegetable on the diet (again, with the exception of lettuce) with an equal amount of any of the following: artichokes, asparagus, broccoli, cabbage, eggplant, sauerkraut, spinach, turnips. Remember, vegetables must be eaten raw, steamed, or boiled. Only salt, pepper, or lemon juice may be used for seasoning.

Egg/meat substitutions. If you cannot eat eggs, you may replace the two eggs at dinner on Day One and the two eggs at lunch on Day Four with four ounces of chicken, *or* two ounces of steak or hamburger.

If your budget won't stretch to accommodate steak and lamb chops, you may replace them with hard-boiled eggs, hamburger, or chicken. At lunch on Day One and at dinner on Day Four, the Four-Day Wonder Diet allows an unspecified amount of steak, which you may replace with as much hamburger or chicken or as many eggs as you need to feel comfortably full and satisfied. To replace the single lamb chop at lunch on Day Two, you may have up to four ounces of hamburger, up to five ounces of chicken, or three hard-boiled eggs.

Tomato substitutions. The tomato in the lettuce and tomato salad at lunch on Day One may be replaced by one green pepper cut into rings or strips, one medium carrot, cut into strips, or two medium pimentos.

For the stewed tomatoes at dinner on Day Three, you may substitute any of the other vegetables on the Four-Day Wonder Diet, or any of the suggested replacements listed in the Vegetable Substitutions section above. If absolutely necessary, the tomato juice at lunch on Day Two and Day Four can be replaced by beef or chicken bouillon.

Fruit substitutions. If you are allergic to grapefruit or apples (and applesauce), you may replace either with the other. Or you may substitute any of the following: three small apricots; one-half medium cantaloupe; one medium nectarine; one small orange; one medium peach; one-half cup fresh cubed pineapple; two small plums; one scant cup strawberries.

Juice substitutions. The unsweetened pineapple juice at dinner on Day Four can be replaced by apple juice. There is no good substitute for prune juice; luckily allergic reactions to prunes are relatively uncommon.

2. *Don't eat* anything *between meals.*

There are *no snacks* on the Four-Day Wonder Diet. None! Even items listed as "free foods" on other diets—foods such as carrot sticks, raw mushrooms, pickles, and boullion—are off limits on this one. And even though you are permitted to have unlimited amounts of certain vegetables at mealtimes, they are not to be "saved," and eaten between meals.

Why is this rule so important? You probably already know from previous attempts at dieting that even a small amount of between-meal eating has a way of opening a whole Pandora's box of potential problems. Whether the snack is celery sticks or an apple . . . it doesn't matter. The very *act* of snacking seems to activate a little voice that whispers, "Come on . . . if this much is okay, then why not a bit more?" The little voice continues to coax, becomes louder and more insistent, and the next thing you know it's SHOUTING for CHOCOLATE CAKE.

Whoever put the Four-Day Wonder Diet together in the first place didn't want to give that little voice a chance to sabotage your chances for success!

Remember, you can have as much as you like—at *mealtimes*—of most of the vegetables on the Four-Day Wonder Diet. The same is true of meat at lunch on Day One and dinner on Day Four, and of chicken at lunch on Day Three. With so much food to fill up on at mealtimes it's quite possible that you will never experience *real* hunger on this diet—at least not the kind of hunger that signals an empty stomach in need of food. However, if you are accustomed to eating between meals, you'll probably feel a compelling urge to snack. This isn't hunger, but habit asserting itself. Try to recognize it for what it is, and don't give in!

If your desire to nibble becomes so intense that it distracts you from work or other activities, give your jaws some exercise by chewing on a stick of sugar-free gum. You'll find lots of other ideas for dealing with real and fake hunger in the chapters that follow.

3. Don't drink alcoholic beverages of any kind.

There are two excellent reasons for avoiding alcohol while you are on the Four-Day Wonder Diet. For one thing, contrary to what some people believe, alcohol *does* contain calories. And, though you don't need to count calories on this diet, you also don't want to add to your daily total. In addition, alcoholic drinks are essentially carbohydrate compounds and have none of the fat-burning potential of the protein foods, which tend to *accelerate* weight loss. In fact, adding carbohydrates to this diet can offset some of the fat-blitzing effects of protein.

Let's also not forget that one of the special properties of alcohol is its capacity for lowering inhibitions. For many people, that's its greatest appeal! But just as one or two drinks might help you feel more at ease in certain situations, they might also lull that part of your mind that keeps you alert and motivated to stick with your diet.

Does all of this mean you have to stand around empty-handed at parties when you're on the Four-Day Wonder Diet? Not at all. But instead of ordering wine or beer or hard liquor, enjoy a tall glass of seltzer with ice and a wedge of lemon or lime. It will give you something to do with your hands, it's refreshing, and it looks so much like a "real" drink that no one but you and the bartender will know that it isn't.

4. Drink plenty of water while you are on the diet.

Aim for eight eight-ounce glasses each day. Water is important because of the increased amounts of protein foods you will be eating. In the complex fat-burning process by which protein is metabolized, more water than usual is drawn from the cells of the body. This water must be replenished. More water is also needed to wash fatty acids, byproducts of the fat-burning process, out of the kidneys.

Don't drink large amounts of water all at one time, however. Instead, have one eight-ounce glass first thing in the morning, one before each meal, one in the middle of the afternoon and one before you go to bed. That's five glasses. Sip the rest at odd intervals throughout the day. (Some dieters discover that sipping at a tall glass of ice water helps assuage the urge to nibble!)

Yes, you probably *will* need to visit the bathroom more often while you are on the Four-Day Wonder Diet. Anticipate and allow for it. The temporary inconvenience will all be forgotten as the pounds begin to disappear. That's a promise!

5. Have as much black coffee or plain tea as you like, but limit diet soda to two twelve-ounce bottles per day.

You may sweeten your coffee or tea with artificial sweetener, but don't add milk, half-and-half, cream, or nondairy creamer.

If you are a very heavy coffee and tea drinker, you might find it helpful to switch to a decaffeinated product, or a caffeine-free herb tea while you are on the Four-Day Wonder Diet. Some coffee and tea lovers, even those with an amazing capacity for downing cup after cup of their favorite beverage without feeling jangled, discover that dieting makes them more vulnerable to caffeine nerves. There is also some evidence that caffeine stimulates the appetite—another good reason to avoid overconsumption of ordinary coffee or tea while you diet.

Do not drink more than the limit of two twelve-ounce bottles of diet soda. Many diet sodas are sweetened with sodium saccharin, and contain ingredients such as sodium benzoate and sodium citrate. As you probably know, sodium and salt are practically synonymous, and any substance that has sodium as part of its name will add to your total daily salt intake. Of course, salt won't make you fat, but excessive amounts can cause the body to retain fluid. This "water weight" can mask true weight loss on a diet.

6. *Eat vegetables raw, steamed, or boiled.*

Though eating raw green beans, squash, and cauliflower might strike you as being unnecessarily Spartan, you may discover that the crispness and subtle flavors of these vegetables uncooked are positively addictive. It's worth a try, at least.

If you'd rather cook your vegetables, steaming or boiling in a small amount of water until just tender are the preferred methods. Do not sauté, fry, or stir-fry vegetables on the Four-Day Wonder Diet.

Naturally, a steamer is the best tool for steaming, but it isn't an absolute must. You could use a metal colander instead. Whichever you use, it should be positioned over a pot of rapidly boiling water. It's important that the steamer or colander be secured so that its bottom is suspended slightly *above,* not in, the water. After adding the vegetables, cover the pot tightly.

To prepare fresh green beans for steaming or boiling, simply rinse them well and break off the ends. You can cook them whole, break them into bite-size pieces, or slice them lengthwise. Steam for about fifteen minutes, or boil for about ten minutes.

To prepare fresh cauliflower, rinse well, remove leaves from the head, cut off the tough part of the stem, then break the head into flowerets. Steam for about eight minutes, or boil for about six minutes.

To prepare summer squash or zucchini, rinse well, cut off stem and blossom ends, then slice into rounds or cut into cubes. Steam for twelve to fifteen minutes, or boil for eight to ten minutes.

7. Broil all meat and chicken.

As you know, calories are not a primary consideration on this diet, but there's no point in adding unnecessarily to the total. Thus, frying and sautéeing are to be avoided because either method of cooking would add small amounts of fat. In proper broiling done on a rack, no extra fat is used and much of the fat contained in the meat itself is liquefied and melts off into the pan below.

Tips on how to buy and broil steak and hamburger. When shopping for steak, avoid those gorgeous prime cuts that are amply marbled with fat. Choice-grade steaks are every bit as delicious though somewhat less tender. They're also quite a bit less expensive, and decidedly less fatty.

To broil a steak, turn oven or range control to "broil" and place meat on a broiler rack. If the steak is about an inch thick, insert broiler pan and rack so that the top of the steak is two to three inches from the heat. A thicker steak should be placed an inch or so farther from the heat. Broil until the top is nicely browned, then turn and finish cooking on the other side. A one-inch steak will take about fifteen minutes to reach the rare stage. A thicker steak will take a few minutes longer.

In buying hamburger, be prepared to pay a bit more than the rock-bottom bargain price. The least expensive hamburger has a relatively high fat content. As cheap hamburger cooks, the fat liquefies; some is absorbed into the meat, the rest melts off, leaving you with much less to eat than you bargained for.

To broil hamburger, shape into patties one inch thick, place on broiler rack and cook about three inches from heat. Broil about six minutes on each side if you like your burgers rare. For medium-well burgers, cook about eight minutes per side.

Tips on how to buy and broil a lamb chop. Selecting a lamb chop is simple. Just look for one with the best ratio of meat to fat and bone.

To broil a chop that is one inch thick, place it on a broiler rack about two inches from the heat. When one side is browned, turn and finish cooking on the other side. Total cooking time should be ten to twelve minutes. To cook a two-inch-thick chop, place it about three inches from the heat. Broil, as above, for about twenty minutes.

Tips on how to buy and broil chicken. In selecting chicken, keep in mind that broilers are somewhat lower in calories than roasters, and that light, or "white" meat has fewer calories than dark.

To broil a chicken, place skin-side down on a broiler rack and insert pan so that the thickest pieces are between four and five inches from the heat. Broil for about fifteen minutes, then turn chicken skin-side up and broil for another fifteen minutes.

8. *Remove all traces of fat from meat and chicken before you eat it.*

If you shop carefully, there won't be much fat on your steak or lamb chop, but there may be some. In trimming it away, you can avoid many unnecessary calories. It is important to remove chicken skin, because most of the fat is in, or just under, the skin. (Some people prefer to strip off the skin before cooking chicken.)

9. Use only salt, pepper, or lemon juice to season food.

No other flavorings, herbs, spices, or condiments are allowed on the Four-Day Wonder Diet. Not even those that are low-cal or no-cal. That means no oil, mayonnaise, or even vinegar on salads. No dietetic salad dressing, either. No margarine or butter on vegetables. No mustard, ketchup, Worcestershire, or other steak sauce on meat.

The idea is to keep meals as plain and simple as possible so that as a dieter you will be focusing less on the pleasure of eating and more on your main objective: losing as many pounds as possible as quickly as possible. The less you fuss with seasonings, the less attention you pay to adjusting flavors so that they are more to your liking, the less inclined you will be to think of food as a source of gratification instead of fuel. If you can get yourself to think of food as fuel, no more, no less—at least while you're dieting—you'll be that much ahead at winning the losing game!

A few words about salt. Use it sparingly. As you know, salt has no calories, so it won't add to your daily total. But as mentioned earlier, excessive use of salt in cooking and seasoning food can increase fluid retention. This in turn can make you weigh more, resulting in a "false" reading on the bathroom scale—and the discouraging feeling that you're getting nowhere fast on your diet. (The loss of up to a pound or so of fat could conceivably be canceled out by the weight of excess fluid retained by the body!) Don't let it happen to you—frustration because of lack of progress is one of the major reasons people go off their diets.

You may be doing yourself a favor in more ways than one by cutting back on salt and high-sodium foods—not just for now, on the Four-Day Wonder Diet, but for always. Many doctors and public health officials have expressed concern about the high per capita salt intake in the United States as it relates to the high incidence of hypertension in our population. These experts encourage almost everyone—dieters and nondieters—to think twice before they reach for the salt shaker.

10. Fill up, but don't overdo it!

There are no quantities or amounts specified for some of the foods on the Four-Day Wonder Diet. Where no limit is given, you may eat as much as you like. If you're like most dieters, you will be looking forward to those meals that include unlimited steak or chicken—it's only natural! However, for best results on the diet, it's important not to go hog wild. You'll end up feeling stuffed and uncomfortable and, probably, a little bit guilty. Though you *will* lose weight on the Four-Day Wonder Diet no matter how much meat and chicken you eat, you'll lose *more* if you eat them in moderation.

"Listen" to your stomach, if your goal is to lose the maximum number of pounds on the Four-Day Wonder Diet. Eat as much as you like, to satisfy your appetite, but don't ignore your tummy when it tells you it's full.

11. Don't stay on the Four-Day Wonder Diet longer than four days.

If you follow the food plan exactly and pay careful attention to all the important dos and don'ts in this chapter, you'll be amazed at the results. You'll feel terrific, too—vibrant, full of energy, ready to take on the world!

Looking back on the four days, you'll wonder at how

the time flew and at how easy it all was in retrospect. You may be tempted, in fact, to extend your losing streak for a week, or more. Don't do it.

There's never been any diet quite like the Four-Day Wonder Diet for losing pounds in a hurry. But the special combination of foods that makes the Four-Day Wonder Diet the best diet ever for short-term weight loss also makes it unsuitable for use over extended periods.

Resume your normal eating habits when you've completed your first round of the Four-Day Wonder Diet. Or, if your goal is to lose additional pounds, switch immediately to a good long-distance diet. If you want to, or need to, you can always come back again to the Four-Day Wonder Diet in a month or six weeks for another round of fast, fabulous weight loss!

FOUR

Diet Countdown: Nine Tips to Make It Easier on Yourself

YOU KNOW ALL ABOUT the basic diet now. You know which foods to eat and in what amounts. You even know how each of the different food groups included in the Four-Day Wonder Diet contributes to fast, no-fail weight loss. Just as important, you know the rules and regulations that make it all work, and why it is important to follow these rules to the letter. In short, you're ready to start your first round of Four-Day Wonder dieting... and lose five, seven, even ten pounds within the next few days.

The tips that follow will get you off to a flying start. They'll minimize problems that can arise on this or *any* diet and help maximize the number of pounds you'll lose. They'll help you sail through the first two days with ease, and make the final two days go like clockwork.

1. Pick an appropriate, convenient time to go on the 4-Day Wonder Diet.

If your motivation is high, you can expect terrific results from the diet *any* time you feel a desire to lose weight.

Still, you can make it even easier on yourself if you plan to diet when your schedule doesn't include a string of parties, luncheons, and other social gatherings where food will be served.

This shouldn't be difficult. One of the great things about the Four-Day Wonder Diet is that it accomplishes in less than a work week what most other diets take two or three times as long to achieve. Since most parties are planned for the weekend, they needn't interfere with your diet. You can lose weight without skipping a beat, where your social life is concerned, if you time your diet to begin on a Monday or Tuesday.

On the other hand, if your job requires you to attend many luncheons or other business-related functions during or after the workday, plan to start the Four-Day Wonder Diet on a Friday. You'll be finished up—and pounds slimmer—by Tuesday. And at worst, you'll have to deal with only two business luncheons.

Eating in restaurants needn't be a problem on the Four-Day Wonder Diet. You can order plain broiled steak or hamburger, chicken or a lamb chop in almost any restaurant. Some ethnic and certain specialty establishments with very limited menus are possible exceptions. These must be avoided until after you've completed the Four-Day Wonder Diet.

2. *Shop ahead.*

The day before you plan to start the diet—and certainly no later than Day One—make a shopping list of every single item you'll need for the full four days, and stock up.

With everything you need safely stashed away in fridge or freezer, you'll never be caught in a situation where, as one dieter put it, "the spirit was willing, but the only thing in the house was spaghetti."

Don't worry about spoilage or buying too much. The vegetables will keep very nicely in a crisper until the end of the four-day period; meat will be safe in the freezer, and if there is anything left over, you can certainly use it up soon after you've completed the diet.

3. Decide how to integrate your diet with family meals.

Obviously, if you live alone you can skip this one. But if you're in charge of cooking for the people you live with— or even if your husband or roommate does most of the cooking—you'll need to make a decision about the evening meal: Should everyone in the household have the same basic food (*yours,* naturally, since your food choices are limited while you are on the diet and theirs are flexible)? Or should an agreement be made to cook two separate, different dinners—one for you, and one for them—while you are on the Four-Day Wonder Diet?

The first option is definitely simplest for everyone. In fact, you may be pleasantly surprised to discover how easily Four-Day Wonder Diet menus can be adapted for family eating. It's only necessary to make a few additions. Here's how it might work:

4-DAY WONDER DIET DINNER		FAMILY DINNER
DAY ONE	Grapefruit	Grapefruit
	2 hard-boiled eggs	Western omelet (or fish)
	Green beans	Green beans (buttered, perhaps)
		Baked potato
		Ice cream
DAY TWO		Tomato juice
		Lamb chops
	Squash and	Squash and

	cauliflower	cauliflower
	Green beans	Green beans
	Unsweetened applesauce	Pound cake topped with unsweetened applesauce
DAY THREE		Vegetable juice
	Hamburger	Hamburger
	Stewed tomatoes	Stewed tomatoes
		Rice
	Prune juice	Fruit cup
DAY FOUR	6 ounces unsweetened pineapple juice	Unsweetened pineapple juice
	Broiled steak	Broiled steak
	Lettuce and tomato salad (no dressing)	Lettuce and tomato salad (with dressing, if desired)
		Julienne potatoes
		Apple tart

As you can see, in each case a starchy vegetable and dessert were added to round out the family version of the Four-Day Wonder Diet meals. On Day Two, when your diet dinner is essentially vegetarian, meat was added to the family meal. (In the example above, it was lamb chops; a logical choice, since a lamb chop is featured on the Four-Day Wonder Diet Day Two lunch menu.) Though your family or housemates might have other preferences with regard to augmenting the Four-Day Wonder Diet, the suggestions above illustrate how easily the meals on this diet can be modified so that even nondieters will enjoy them.

4. If you don't already own one, invest in a good bathroom scale.

Even if your weight problem is a relatively small one, and your primary goal is simply to sleek down enough to fit into a favorite figure-flattering dress or neatly tailored pants, an accurate scale is important. Watching the needle on the scale register your weight loss—one, two, even three pounds each day—is exhilarating and will help reinforce your will to stay on the Four-Day Wonder Diet. Not only that, starting with Day One a daily weigh-in is an integral part of the diet process, since you are going to chart your progress in a journal. (More about this journal in a moment.)

An old, cheap scale that has been exposed for years to bathroom humidity, which can cause interior rusting, may not be sensitive enough to accurately register losses of a pound or less. (It might give you a ballpark figure, but that's not good enough when you are dieting.)

The most accurate weighing devices of all are the balance-type scales that you have used in the doctor's office. These are more expensive than the ordinary spring-type bathroom scales, and because they take up more space, they're not as convenient for use in a small bathroom. However, scales that operate on the balance principle are practically indestructible. Humidity and rust won't affect their accuracy. And if you want to keep careful track of your weight—not just now, when you're planning to diet, but for all the years to come—one of these scales would be a good investment.

If you'd rather stick with the more familiar spring-type bathroom scale, buy one, if possible, in the medium-to-high price range. Spending a few dollars more for a really good quality scale will be worth it in terms of its greater sensitivity to small variations in weight.

Even a good new spring-type scale should be checked for accuracy every so often. The easiest way to do this is to place a "standard" weight—such as a five- or ten-pound bag of sugar or flour, or a small barbell or exercise weight—on the scale. Then adjust the scale, if necessary, so that the needle points to the five- or ten-pound mark.

5. Keep a diet journal.

You'll need a notebook, to be used for this purpose only. (A pocket-size spiral notebook that fits easily into your purse would be ideal.) In your journal, you will record the date you begin the Four-Day Wonder Diet, as well as your weight first thing in the morning on Day One, and on each of the following four mornings. On days when you expect to be away from home for lunch or dinner, you should also copy into your journal the Four-Day Wonder Diet menus for that day so that you'll know exactly what to order at coffee shop or restaurant.

Many dieters report that keeping track of the number of pounds lost each day and entering their new weight in a journal adds a new dimension to the weight loss process. Will power actually builds as the pounds melt away, and dieting becomes less a chore and a bore, more an exciting competition with the self. Like these others, you may find yourself looking forward with anticipation to recording your progress each day—even if you always went out of your way to *avoid* a confrontation with the scale in the past!

Some people also find it helpful to use their journal as a kind of confidante. For example, one woman who has been highly successful with the Four-Day Wonder Diet often jots notes of encouragement to herself in the morning. She reads these private pep talks later on in the day to keep herself motivated. And when she's tempted to eat something she shouldn't, she opens her journal and makes a list of all the reasons for staying on the diet: She'll look more attractive, she'll *feel* more attractive, her clothes will fit better, she'll respect herself for accomplishing what she set out to do, and so on. Just making that list takes her mind off the forbidden food and helps her refocus on the goal of blitzing off pounds.

6. Don't talk about it!

The less you say about your diet, the better. Believe it! Even your closest relatives and dearest friends, the people who want nothing but the best for you, will soon be bored to tears if you insist on giving them a blow-by-blow account of the food you are eating (or not eating), your hunger pangs (or the surprising lack of them), your heroic struggles against food temptations, et cetera, et cetera. The truth of the matter is that while what you experience as you diet is of major, all-consuming interest to *you*, it is simply not that fascinating to others.

Then there is the fact that talking about your diet will often elicit a response that undercuts your will to stay on the diet. Well-meaning people may express surprise when you tell them that you're trying to lose weight, especially if you're not really *fat* and only want to take off a few pounds. Of course, it's flattering to be told that you look just fine the way you are, and that you don't need to lose an ounce. But it can also weaken your resolve.

There is also the possibility that those you take into your confidence will be critical of the Four-Day Wonder Diet. They may even attempt to seduce you into following their own favorite program. This, too, can be demoralizing.

It will be easier if you talk about your diet as little as possible while you are on it. Afterward, when everyone marvels at how great you look, crow all you like about how quickly you lost *all those pounds*. (And don't be surprised if the very people who tried to get you to follow *their* diet suddenly start asking for more information about *yours!*)

7. *Try to be more active while you are on the 4-Day Wonder Diet—and afterward as well.*

It was emphasized in an earlier chapter that you should not start any new program of strenuous physical activity while you are on the diet. However, assuming that you are in good health, there's no reason why you shouldn't begin to exercise *moderately*. Increased activity will enhance feelings of well-being and help the pounds melt off even more quickly.

It is true that many diet experts are skeptical about the value of exercise in a weight reduction program. They point to the fact that in order to burn off a pound of fat—thirty-five hundred calories—a woman weighing 120 pounds would have to run for slightly more than five hours! (In running, a person weighing 120 pounds will burn off approximately seven hundred calories per hour; a heavier person will burn calories more rapidly.) What they often neglect to mention is the *cumulative* effect of increased physical activity.

Though it is certainly true that you have to run for about five hours to burn off a pound of fat, you don't have to run for five hours at a time! You could run an hour a day for five days. Or half an hour a day for ten days. Or fifteen minutes a day for twenty days. You don't even have to *run*. (Indeed, you certainly should *not* embark on an ambitious running program if you're not already in tiptop shape.) You could walk briskly, for example. In fact, if you took a brisk half-hour walk twice a day for four days, you'd burn off an extra twelve hundred calories whether you were on a diet or eating normally.

Since upping your level of physical activity increases

the number of calories your body burns off, exercise will *enhance* the results you get on the Four-Day Wonder Diet, or any diet for that matter. It's important to make the point that exercise isn't crucial to the success of the Four-Day Wonder Diet—you'll lose up to two-and-a-half pounds a day, exercise or no exercise. But by being more active you can insure that you will lose as much as it is possible for you to lose, given your height, current weight, body build, and age. (For more on exercise, see Chapter Eleven.)

8. Don't binge on the day before you start the 4-Day Wonder Diet.

There's an almost irresistible impulse to go all out on the eve of starting a new diet. It's utterly understandable: The dieter wants to have one last food fling before settling down to a long, drawn-out period of self-denial.

However, with the Four-Day Wonder Diet, there *is* no long, drawn-out period of self-denial. It's over and done with in less than week. And though you can stuff yourself to your heart's content on the day before and *still* end up with a gratifying net loss at the end of the four days, chances are you will be even more delighted with the results if you eat normally the day before you start the diet.

Day-before gorging will put you at a disadvantage because your body will have to deal with the excess before it can get down to the serious business of burning off fat on Day One. To reiterate: If you *really* want to lose as many pounds as possible on the Four-Day Wonder Diet, don't go off on a wild food rampage the day before.

9. Cultivate a "losing" frame of mind.

Even if you've had only minimal success with other diets in the past, you *will* lose more pounds, more quickly, with the Four-Day Wonder Diet than you ever thought possible, if you follow the diet exactly.

Of course, to follow any diet exactly is easier said than done. But one thing is certain: Confidence in yourself and in the effectiveness of your diet can work wonders. That's why it's so important to put yourself in a winning—or, more precisely, losing—frame of mind right from the very beginning. If you're pretty sure you'll be able to stay on the diet for four days, you probably will. If you *know* you can, success is practically guaranteed!

The Four-Day Wonder Diet *works*. It has worked for others time and again, and it will work for you. All you have to do is give this incredible diet a chance... and let the food and your body do the rest.

DAY ONE

BREAKFAST   *½ grapefruit*
                Black coffee or plain tea

LUNCH   *Broiled steak*
                Lettuce and tomato salad, no
                    dressing
                1 apple

DINNER   *2 hard-boiled eggs*
                Green beans
                ½ grapefruit

FIVE

The 4-Day Wonder Diet: Day One

READY TO START your first round of the Four-Day Wonder Diet? Terrific! In the next four chapters—one for each day of the diet—you'll find dozens of suggestions, tips, tricks, and techniques to guide you every step of the way through the entire cycle. As you will see, some of the suggestions apply to Four-Day Wonder dieting only. Others will be equally helpful in subsequent dieting, should you decide to switch immediately to a long-term weight loss program after you've lost initial pounds and inches on the Four-Day Wonder Diet.

Read through the entire four chapters now, before you actually begin Day One. Taken all together, these chapters will provide a useful overview. They'll also clue you in, in advance, on what you can expect to experience on each day of the Four-Day Wonder Diet, and tip you off on how to handle potential problems. Then, each morning as you proceed with the diet, turn again to the appropriate chapter for a refresher course.

Important reminder! If you haven't done so already, check with your doctor now, before you start Day One of the Four-Day Wonder Diet. Don't be surprised if he or she does not express enormous enthusiasm for this diet. Do point out that you do not intend to use it for long periods of time, and that you will be finished with it in a quick four days.

DAY ONE...WAKE UP, WEIGH, AND MEASURE

Good morning! Summer, winter...rain or shine...it's a great day to get started. Weighing in is first thing on the agenda. Don't drink or eat anything yet. Don't even brush your teeth! Go into the bathroom, take off your clothes (everything, including bedroom slippers), urinate, then step on the scales. This is your starting weight and should be recorded in your diet journal.

Though it isn't a must, you might also find it helpful to measure yourself, too. (You'll certainly want a record of your dimensions if you are planning to start a long-distance diet for additional weight loss when you've finished with the Four-Day Wonder Diet.) You will need a tape measure for accurate measuring. In using it, pull it tightly enough to draw up any slack, but not so tightly that it depresses the flesh.

To get an accurate *bust* measurement, the tape should encircle your upper back and breasts at nipple level.

Measure your *waist* at the level of greatest indentation. (Stomach measurement for men should be taken at belly button level.)

Measure around the widest part of your *hips*.

Measure your *thighs* midway between the knee and hip joints.

WATER BREAK

Remember, you are going to drink eight eight-ounce glasses of water today: one before each meal, one at mid-afternoon, one at bedtime. The rest can be sipped with meals or at odd moments throughout the day. As mentioned earlier, drinking plenty of water is important on the Four-Day Wonder Diet. It will help your kidneys wash away the fatty acids that are the byproducts of speeded-up fat metabolism. Even though your diet is just beginning and your body hasn't yet shifted into highest fat-burning gear, you should have a glass of water now, before breakfast, to establish the habit of getting more fluids into your body.

As the diet progresses, you will discover for yourself another excellent reason for drinking water before meals. Because it takes up room in your stomach, water will contribute to a feeling of comfortable fullness and you will leave the table feeling more satisfied, with less food.

Tip: Instead of plain, cold water, try hot water with a slice of lemon. The lemon adds a bright wakeup taste, and many people find that warm liquids are more satisfying than cold.

MINI-WORKOUT!

Before you get into the shower, try this to burn off a few extra calories: Switch on the radio. Dial around until you find some peppy, upbeat music. Now run in place for sixty seconds. Keep your knees flexed and pump hard with your arms for maximum benefits.

BREAKFAST

Today, as every day on the Four-Day Wonder Diet, breakfast is one-half grapefruit and black coffee or plain tea. Don't skip it. Even if you normally go without breakfast, you should eat in the morning while you are on this diet. Lunch is a long way off, and snacking is not allowed on the Four-Day Wonder Diet.

BONUS IDEAS FOR ADDITIONAL CALORIE BURNOFF

Anything you can do to increase your level of physical activity will help you lose more weight on a diet. Anything! Do you take a bus to work in the morning? If so, why not walk—briskly—*past* your regular stop and board the bus two or three blocks down the line? You could do the same at the other end: Instead of getting off at your usual stop, signal the driver to let you off one or two blocks early, then walk briskly the rest of the way to your office.

Another idea: If you're in good health, climbing stairs is terrific exercise. If your office is on the tenth floor, get off the elevator on the eighth and walk up the rest of the way. Walking down stairs won't burn off as many calories as climbing up, but it will burn off more than riding in the elevator.

Tip: For even greater calorie burnoff, cultivate the habit of doing things the hard way. The possibilities are practically endless. Starting today, for example, you could take a walk down the hall to speak to a co-worker instead of using the office intercom. You could reach up high to stow a file on a top shelf instead of tossing it onto a lower one. You could use a crank-type, hand-powered pencil sharpener instead of the electric kind. Individually, none of these small exertions will burn off more than just a few extra calories, but over a period of days, they add up.

DAY ONE LUNCH

(Reminder: Have a tall glass of water a few minutes before you sit down to eat.)

For lunch today you're going to have broiled steak, as much as you like; plain lettuce and tomato salad, again as much as you like; and an apple. Eating at home will pose no problems. If you're going to be away from home at lunchtime, you can pack food and eat at your desk. Make sure you also pack a fork and a good steak knife.

If you'd rather not pack a lunch, look for a restaurant or coffee shop that caters to an ordinary lunchtime crowd. (Stay away from Chinese, Italian, and—obviously—vegetarian places that do not offer plain broiled meat.) If you don't see steak on the menu order a steak sandwich. Don't eat the bread. And, as discreetly as possible, scrape away any sauce, fried onions, or other garnish served with the sandwich. Be sure to tell the waitress to hold the dressing on your salad. If you can't get an apple at the restaurant, buy one at a grocery or deli and eat it at your desk back at the office.

WHAT ABOUT MIDAFTERNOON SLUMP?

Many people, not just dieters, feel less energetic a few hours after eating lunch. Often, this feeling of lassitude is accompanied by a craving for something to eat. Hunger may be insistent even on those days when lunch was a relatively elaborate, high-calorie affair. Late-afternoon lassitude is usually associated with lowered levels of sugar in the blood. However, strangely enough, you may discover that midafternoon slump is *not* a problem today, or on any of the Four-Day Wonder Diet days.

How come? Because lunches on the Four-Day Wonder Diet are all low in carbohydrates and high in protein— higher in protein, perhaps, than the lunches you have been eating all along. And protein, though it is slower to elevate blood sugar levels than carbohydrates, tends to keep blood sugar levels *higher*, for *longer* periods of time.

If you do notice a let-down feeling in the afternoon, take time out for a tea or coffee break. The caffeine in either should perk you up and give you just enough of the bounce you need to get through comfortably until dinner.

DAY ONE DINNER

Dinner today is two boiled eggs, plus all the green beans you want, and half a grapefruit.

If you have a choice, eat dinner at home. But if you *must* dine out at a restaurant, all is not lost. The biggest obstacle to staying on the Four-Day Wonder Diet, or any diet, in a restaurant is the dieter's own self-consciousness about ordering obviously low-cal food. What so many dieters forget when they're sitting there in a restaurant wondering whether they dare order diet food is that waiters—especially the waiters in better restaurants—are accustomed to all kinds of special requests for food not listed on the menu. Can you imagine the high-powered executive or diplomat or show biz personality hesitating to order food recommended by a doctor for ulcers, hypertension, a heart—or weight—problem? No, of course not. Then why should *you* be reluctant to order in accordance with *your* needs?

As for your dinner partners, chances are they've all been dieters, too, at one time or another. They *know* what it's like and they'll probably be supportive. And if someone *does* try to talk you into eating something that is not on your diet? Simply shrug and decline, firmly but with a smile. Then change the subject. It's that easy!

BEDTIME

Congratulations. You did it! You breezed through Day One of the Four-Day Wonder Diet, and you're probably feeling slimmer and fitter already. You're also probably surprised at how easy it was to stay on the diet. Make up your mind now that you'll be equally successful on Days Two, Three, and Four. Results will begin to show soon—on the scale and in the fit of your clothes. In just a few days, you'll be finished with the diet... feeling marvelous and *pounds* thinner!

DAY TWO

BREAKFAST   *½ grapefruit*
             Black coffee or plain tea

LUNCH   *1 lamp chop*
             Lettuce, no dressing
             6 ounces tomato juice

DINNER   *Squash and cauliflower, steamed*
                 or raw
             Green beans
             Unsweetened applesauce

SIX

The 4-Day Wonder Diet: Day Two

IF YOU FELT GREAT last night before you went to bed, it's probably nothing to the way you feel this morning upon awakening: lighter, bursting with energy, full of confidence, and eager to get on with the day and the diet that will pare off up to ten pounds in the next seventy-two hours!

Right now, before you do anything else, reach for your diet journal and give yourself the congratulations you deserve—in writing. Now is also the time to recommit yourself to following the Four-Day Wonder Diet to the letter today, tomorrow, and the next day.

WEIGHING IN

Get undressed, step on the scales...and don't be discouraged if you weigh the same today as you did yesterday. It's important to keep in mind that no matter how slim and fit you *feel* this morning, your body began its shift into high fat-burning gear only yesterday, and it is still too early for dramatic results. Although some people *do* drop a pound by the morning of Day Two, most don't. In fact, a few dieters actually weigh *more* on Day Two. This is because their bodies have not yet adjusted to the greatly increased fluid intake of the day before.

It's important enough to be repeated: Don't allow yourself to be demoralized if you find that you have gained a small amount of weight since yesterday. The additional half pound or so is *not* fat but water, and will vanish as soon as your body's water balance has been reestablished.

Above all, don't neglect to drink the full eight eight-ounce glasses of water today.

MINI-WORKOUT!

Were you able to run in place for a full sixty seconds yesterday without feeling winded? If so, try for ninety seconds today. Remember, keep your knees flexed and pump your arms. (Stop immediately if you begin to feel uncomfortable; ninety seconds isn't much, but it's a lot if you are unaccustomed to this kind of exercise.)

Calorie Burnoff Bonus: If you have a few extra minutes this morning, why not tune in to one of the A.M. aerobics shows on television after you've warmed up with a minute or so of running in place? You shouldn't attempt a full half-hour workout if you've been leading a sedentary life for the last few months. However, if you are young and in basic good health, two or three minutes of not-too-vigorous aerobics should be energizing and beneficial in terms of additional calorie burnoff.

BREAKFAST AND LUNCH

Breakfast today as always is one-half grapefruit and black coffee or plain tea.

Lunch is one lamb chop, lettuce with no dressing, and six ounces of tomato juice.

HOW TO GET MORE BANG FOR THE BITE

It's entirely possible that you will *never* feel hungry on the Four-Day Wonder Diet—-or at least not hungry in the literal sense of the word. But you might feel unsatisfied, because while you are on the diet your food choices will be limited and you will be eating nothing between meals.

There's no question that staying on this or any diet is easier when you have a sense of complete physical and psychological satisfaction after meals. Over the years, behavioral scientists have developed a number of techniques that dieters can use to get more satisfaction from less food. More bang for the bite, in other words!

Eat slowly. Many people eat as though they're in a competition to see how fast they can polish off the meal in front of them. In company, they're the first to finish; alone, it's as though they're trying to shave milliseconds off their own best eating time. They don't take time to taste. They chew only as much as is necessary to get the food down without choking. Since the stomach takes about twenty minutes to register satiety, it's no wonder that fast eaters often reach the end of a meal—even a fairly big one—still wanting more.

Naturally, you will be eager to fill up after not eating

for several hours. But try to keep in mind when you sit down at the table that you will ultimately feel *more* satisfaction if you take your time and taste, chew, and swallow as slowly and deliberately as possible.

If fast eating is a habit, these tricks should help you slow down:

—Take two or three sips of water, seltzer, or diet soda between bites of food.

—Place your knife and fork or spoon back on your plate after each bite; don't pick them up again until you are ready for the next bite.

—Chew your food *thoroughly;* don't swallow until it has been completely liquefied.

—If you are dining with others, pace yourself, so that you are the last one finished. If you are alone, be a clock-watcher; try to stretch meals out to a full half hour.

—Don't eat unless, or until, you are properly seated at a table. Sitting down on a chair, at a table, with place-mat, napkin, plates, and silverware, sends important signals to your brain—and indirectly to your stomach—that a "real" meal is on the way. Food eaten while you are standing at the kitchen counter, or peering into the refrigerator, or driving in your car, or walking down the street, sends "snack" signals. And though food eaten while standing or on the run might be every bit as filling and nutritious as food eaten at a table, it won't deliver the same full measure of physical and psychological satisfaction.

Even if it means waiting an extra hour or so, delay eating until you can sit down to enjoy your meal at home or in a restaurant. The wait may be uncomfortable, but it won't hurt you. In fact, it could do you a lot of good! Discovering that you *can* wait will add to your store of confidence in your ability to stick to a diet. It's proof positive that you are in control and that you can shape up with the best of them!

Tip: On the days when you decide to have lunch at your desk, make an effort to create a pleasant, table-like setting. Clear away files and notebooks, spread a napkin to act as a placemat, use a real knife and fork instead of plastic.

—Don't combine eating with other activities. When your mind is focused elsewhere—on a book or newspaper, the television, a crossword puzzle, for example—chewing and swallowing become reflexive rather than deliberate and food satisfaction is necessarily diminished. When food is eaten without full awareness, the result can be "phantom hunger"—the nagging feeling of having missed the meal you have in fact just finished! Nondieters can deal with phantom hunger by raiding the fridge for leftovers. But that's taboo on the Four-Day Wonder Diet.

By focusing on eating instead of dividing your attention between it and some other activity, you'll never have to deal with the phantom hunger that can be a major stumbling block on any diet. You'll be in a stronger position to lose the maximum number of pounds on the Four-Day Wonder Diet.

NOW, ABOUT THOSE BEANS!

As you *must* have noticed by now, green beans are featured prominently in three of the Four-Day Wonder Diet menus: You had them first at dinner on Day One. You will have them again today, at dinner. You will have them once again, at lunch, on Day Four.

Most people have no trouble with this good-tasting, vitamin- and fiber-rich, extremely low-calorie vegetable. But eating large amounts of green beans sometimes does pose a minor problem for a few. That problem is gas, and the noisy stomach and bloating that often go along with it.

If you were annoyed by gas yesterday, try preparing green beans for today's dinner in the following gas-less way: An hour before cooking them, soak the beans in a pot of cool water to which you have added a handful of baking soda. (Stir first, to dissolve the baking soda.) There should be enough water in the pot to cover the beans. After soaking, rinse the beans thoroughly, then steam or boil as usual.

Tip: If gas is a frequent problem for you —beans or no beans, diet or no diet—try walking or engaging in some other form of mild physical activity after dinner instead of remaining sedentary. (Also, because swallowing air is another cause of the discomfort associated with gas, chew your food slowly, with your mouth closed, and sip beverages rather than gulp them.)

DAY TWO DINNER

Today you will have as much as you like of steamed or raw cauliflower and squash, green beans, and unsweetened applesauce. Of all the Four-Day Wonder Diet dinners, this one is the most Spartan, because of its vegetarian nature. Meat and other animal protein foods, such as eggs, literally stay with you longer than fruits and vegetables. Think about it a moment. Haven't you noticed that you feel fuller for a longer time after a meal that included three or four ounces of meat than after a meatless meal? (In fact, it's the relative meatlessness of so much Chinese food that accounts for that proverbial surge of hunger that you experience an hour or so after you eat it!)

If you're *ever* going to feel hungry on the Four-Day Wonder Diet, it will be this evening, in the hours before bedtime. Forewarned is forearmed. Try to stay busy to keep your mind off food. If possible, get out of the house and into a food-free environment.

This would be a perfect night to go to a movie, for example. (No popcorn, remember!) Better yet, if you belong to a gym or health club, this would be a great time to drop in for a workout on the machines, or a few laps in the pool. If the stores are open, why not go shopping? (There's nothing like trying on new clothes to steel yourself for staying on a diet.) Or you could take a long, long walk. In a pinch, get in the car and just *drive!*

Don't let a little hunger throw you now. If you do indeed feel hungry, it only means that your body has been accustomed to more food than you gave it today; it's a sure sign that the Four-Day Wonder Diet is doing exactly what you want it to do.

BATH THERAPY

When a persistent craving for food threatens to keep you awake at the end of the day, there's nothing like taking off your clothes and settling into a long, lulling bath. Relaxing in a warm tub has a way of easing much of the tension and fretfulness associated with an empty tummy. Just as important, getting undressed and then soaping, rinsing, and toweling yourself dry will put you in closer touch, literally, with your body. And a long, critical gaze at yourself in a full-length mirror before slipping into your nightgown should banish any thoughts you might have about giving up. It's a strategy that rarely fails. Whether you want to lose just a little weight or a lot, one of the best ways to reaffirm your commitment to getting into super shape is to focus on your body at bathtime.

BEDTIME

You're almost halfway through the Four-Day Wonder Diet now. Your body is in high fat-burning gear, and the marvelous results will soon be evident. For many dieters, Day Two is the most difficult, but you've come through with flying colors. Good for you!

DAY THREE

BREAKFAST	*½ grapefruit* *Black coffee or plain tea*
LUNCH	*Broiled chicken* *Lettuce and celery salad, no dressing* *1 apple*
DINNER	*Hamburger patty* *Stewed tomatoes* *6 ounces prune juice*

SEVEN

The 4-Day Wonder Diet: Day Three

MORE CONGRATULATIONS are in order—you're over the hump! Today you will start the second half of the Four-Day Wonder Diet cycle. Like so many dieters on the initial round of the diet, you probably discovered that the first half was easier by far than you expected it to be. You breezed through Day One; you stood up to any hunger pangs resulting from Day Two's meatless dinner. Now you're wondering whether you'll fare as well on Days Three and Four.

Good news! For most dieters it's all downhill coasting from here. Except for breakfast, there are no more low-protein meals. Lunches and dinners for the next two days will supply you with more than enough animal protein to keep you satisfied and full of energy, with none of the draggy, downbeat feelings—not to mention the irritability—that are the unintended consequences of so many other very low-calorie reducing diets. You can look forward to feeling better and better as the pounds melt away.

WEIGHING IN

Many dieters are *thrilled* when they undress and step on the scale first thing in the morning on Day Three. Some weigh in at three, four, or even five pounds less than their starting weight!

But for a few others, the needle on the scale still has not budged. Their bodies are somewhat slower in adjusting to the Four-Day Wonder Diet eating.

It's impossible to predict with any degree of accuracy how fast, and ultimately how much, any individual will lose on a particular weight loss regimen. It was pointed out in Chapter One that your height and build, your present degree of overweight, your age, and the amount of exercise you get will all influence the number of pounds you lose. (The taller and bigger-boned you are, the fatter you are, the younger you are, and the more active you are, the more pounds you can expect to lose on the Four-Day Wonder Diet.) But those aren't the only factors influencing how quickly or slowly weight loss will show up on the scale.

For women, the time of month can be critical. As you know, there is a tendency for the body to retain more water before and during a menstrual period. And when water is retained instead of released and excreted with urine, it will show up on the scale as pounds *not* lost—even though the fat stores of your body are rapidly being depleted.

Remember that salt intake is another factor that can interfere with accurate measurement of fat lost on a diet. Oversalting foods, or eating food that is naturally high in sodium or has been prepared with large amounts of high-sodium additives, can cause your body to hold on to water, sometimes enough water to register on the scale, partially offsetting your true fat loss!

You can't do anything about the time of month. But you *can* cut back on salt if, upon looking back at your eating pattern during the past two days, you decide that you might have been adding too much to your food.

You can also make an effort to burn off more calories by being more active. Some dieters find that even a relatively mild workout has the effect of "shaking loose" a pound or so. Of course, any weight lost after a short workout would be mostly water, in the form of perspiration, since we know that it would be necessary to exercise very vigorously for several hours to burn off a pound of *fat*. Never mind. Moderate exercise *still* puts you way ahead. The extra activity will burn away a few extra calories. The water you lose through perspiration will help restore your body's water balance. And the weight loss that shows up on the scale will boost your morale and help you stay motivated.

However, though exercise is always a good idea, it isn't essential to losing pounds on the Four-Day Wonder Diet. Sticking to the diet *is*. Even if you're one of the few who by Day Three haven't yet seen results on the bathroom scale, stay with it. Some people lose quickly, starting from the very beginning; others show practically no loss until they weigh in on the morning after Day Four. Then, suddenly, they're several pounds lighter! Whichever weight loss pattern is yours, you *will* lose more pounds than you ever thought possible by the time you've completed the cycle!

WATER REMINDER

With all the talk about how water retained by the body can show up on the scale and partially mask true fat loss, you may be tempted to compensate by drinking less than the full eight eight-ounce glasses of water called for by the diet. This is not a good idea. Now that your body is in high fat-burning gear, you need lots of fluids to help flush fatty acids out of your kidneys. Keep drinking that water!

DAY THREE LUNCH

Today you will have lettuce and celery salad with no dressing, broiled chicken, and an apple.

You'll probably be most interested in that chicken, since it represents the first stick-to-your-ribs animal protein food you've had since lunch yesterday. Enjoy! But at the same time, do be sure to fill up on the salad. (If you're in a restaurant, why not order a second helping of salad?)

On the Four-Day Wonder Diet, salad and other vegetables are stressed, among other reasons, because they provide bulk: What Grandma used to call "roughage," and what now more frequently goes under the name "fiber." (So much has been made of bran and whole grains as sources of fiber that it's easy to forget that many vegetables supply good amounts of this valuable substance.) Bulk, of course, is important in preventing constipation, which can be a terrible nuisance to the dieter. In fact, one of the major valid criticisms of the popular protein-only diets is that they're so low in bulk that the dieter becomes vulnerable to the discomfort and lethargy (even headaches) associated with constipation. That won't happen on the Four-Day Wonder Diet if you do what Grandma always said to do and "eat up all your veggies!"

Tip: Eat vegetables first. This will insure that you won't be too full for them later in the meal and will also take some of the edge off your appetite for the higher-calorie meat, chicken, or egg course of the Four-Day Wonder Diet meals.

SPECIAL DAY THREE NON-FOOD STRESS RELIEF TECHNIQUES

Hunger isn't a problem for most people on the Four-Day Wonder Diet. However, the need for "food soothing" can be troublesome, especially for dieters who have learned to rely on food and eating to relieve stress, help calm nerves, and reduce tension. If you're one of them, you might discover that you feel an increased need for food soothing now when you are a couple of days into the diet, a routine has been established, and some of the newness of the regimen has worn off.

The following non-food stress relievers will keep you on the straight and narrow and help you deal with tension better than any chocolate chip cookie yet invented!

—Deep breathing. When you feel the need for food soothing, hold everything. Sit or stand up straight and take several deep breaths. Inhale slowly through your nose; hold your breath for an instant; then exhale slowly through your mouth. There's no need to gasp, or puff out your chest. Simply breathe in and out a bit more slowly and deeply than you do ordinarily. If you do it properly, you can benefit from calming deep breathing anytime, anywhere, without calling undue attention to yourself.

You may recognize this deep-breathing technique as

the same one used by actors and other performing artists to calm jitters before going onstage to face an audience. It works for them. It will work for you, too. The effects are only temporary, of course. But you will discover that taking several deep breaths when temptation threatens to get the better of you can ease tension long enough to give you a chance to collect yourself and get your priorities back in order.

—Positive picturing. For this, you'll need to be alone for five minutes or so. If you're at home when a desperate need for food soothing strikes, go into your bedroom and close the door. If you're at work, find an empty office. If you're in a restaurant or visiting at someone's home, you can always retreat to the bathroom.

First, sit or lie down in the most comfortable position you can manage. Then close your eyes and concentrate on relaxing all of your muscles, from the top of your head down to your toes. (To release tension from facial muscles, tighten them first by grimacing hard, then relax, letting your jaw hang slack.)

With your eyes still closed, take ten deep, slow breaths. Inhale through your nose; hold for an instant; then exhale through your mouth. Try to make your mind blank. By the time you've counted to ten, you should be thoroughly relaxed and rag-doll limp.

Now spend a few minutes visualizing images of yourself, reed-slim, looking absolutely marvelous, doing something you've always dreamed of. Maybe it's starring on Broadway, or accepting a Nobel Prize, or achieving the admiration of someone you love. Make the fantasy as vivid and detailed as you can. Lose yourself in it completely.

Back in the real world again, you will find that your need for food soothing has diminished, or even disappeared! Positive picturing has been effective for other dieters. Try it once, and you will find yourself relying on it for non-food stress relief whenever tension threatens to get the better of you!

DAY THREE DINNER

Today you will have a hamburger patty and unlimited stewed tomatoes, plus six ounces of prune juice. The prune juice, like all of the fruits and vegetables included on the Four-Day Wonder Diet lunch and dinner menus, helps guard against constipation. Drink it down!

BEDTIME

You did it again. You're almost home free. One more day to go and you will have completed your first round of the Four-Day Wonder Diet, a more vibrant and attractive, sleeked-down, shaped-up version of the you who started the diet only three short days ago!

DAY FOUR

BREAKFAST   *½ grapefruit*
             Black coffee or plain tea

LUNCH   *2 hard-boiled eggs*
             Green beans
             6 ounces tomato juice

DINNER   *Broiled steak*
             Lettuce and tomato salad, no
                 dressing
             6 ounces unsweetened pineapple
                 juice

EIGHT

The 4-Day Wonder Diet: Day Four

WELCOME TO YOUR FINAL DAY on the Four-Day Wonder Diet. Like so many others who have followed the diet to its conclusion, you probably woke up in a mood that is nothing short of triumphant! You may have that heady, "nothing-can-stop-me-now" feeling, the elation of a winner on a roll. And for the best reason in the world: You *are* a winner. You've earned that natural high!

The last thing anyone would want to do at this point is burst your balloon. Nevertheless, you may need to be reminded now that although the end is in sight, it's not all over ... yet. To lose the maximum number of pounds on the Four-Day Wonder Diet, you must stay on the diet for another twenty-four hours.

Today shouldn't be difficult. Your body has become accustomed to the rhythms of the diet. You've proved to yourself that you don't need to eat between meals to function—and in fact thrive. You know for a fact that you are capable of mastering the urge to splurge when you put your mind to it. Your confidence in yourself has grown by leaps and bounds over the past three days, and that, more than anything else, will see you through to the end of the Four-Day Wonder Diet cycle.

WEIGHING IN

Get undressed and step on the scale. The result of today's weigh-in should be exciting. For some dieters, the most dramatic loss of weight occurs between Day Three and Day Four, and the biggest drop in pounds shows up on the scale this morning. (Many people discover that they lose more pounds by Day Four—after only three days on the Four-Day Wonder Diet—than in two weeks of any other diet they have tried in the past!) Record the new weight in your diet journal. As you do, keep in mind that no matter how pleased you are with the number that you write in today, it does not represent the ultimate accounting of all your efforts. The *final* results of the Four-Day Wonder Diet eating won't be in until you weigh yourself first thing tomorrow morning.

DAY FOUR LUNCH

Today's lunch is two hard-boiled eggs, all the green beans you feel like eating, and a six-ounce glass of tomato juice. Start off, as always, with a pre-meal "cocktail" of hot or icy-cold water, flavored with a slice of lemon if you prefer. For maximum food satisfaction, chew thoroughly and eat slowly, pausing as long as possible between bites.

THE DAY FOUR BOREDOM FACTOR
AND HOW TO DEAL WITH IT

By now you've no doubt come to recognize that hunger isn't a major problem on the Four-Day Wonder Diet. (Nor, strangely enough, is hunger a primary cause for lack of success on many other reducing diets.) Though people often *think* they feel hungry when they are dieting, on reflection they usually realize that cravings for food have less to do with an empty stomach than with other factors: Habit is one. (Think of it! If you have, for example, eaten a cinnamon bun at coffee break day after day for the last six months, of course you will miss the bun when you don't eat it!) The need for food soothing is also often interpreted as hunger. And so is boredom!

By Day Four, boredom may be the biggest obstacle to successfully completing the Four-Day Wonder Diet cycle. There are two kinds of boredom to be aware of: One is boredom with the limited variety of food you have been eating. The other is boredom with the constant need to maintain self-discipline.

On the Four-Day Wonder Diet, food boredom may be tied in with a craving for carbohydrates. (Conversely, if you were on a diet that is high in carbohydrates but low in protein, you'd probably experience an increased desire for *protein* foods as the days went by.) Even people who do not ordinarily lust after foods such as pasta and rice, breads and cereals—all forbidden on the Four-Day Wonder Diet—may find themselves with a growing urge for these foods on Day Four. The newly discovered passion for macaroni or mashed potatoes is utterly natural, utterly predictable. It arises in part as a reaction to the basic sameness of the food you've been eating. It can also be viewed as your body's way of asserting its need for a balanced diet, consisting of a wider variety of foods.

Does that mean you should heed your body's call to abandon the diet, and run out for a carbohydrate fix? The answer is yes, in the long run, but no, not today. Aside from the craving for starchy foods, you are probably feeling wonderful, full of energy, pleased with yourself and your progress. And assuming that's the case, there's no reason in the world why you shouldn't stick it out until tomorrow.

In fact, if you want to get maximum weight loss benefits from the Four-Day Wonder Diet, you *must* complete the cycle. If you're healthy, feel good, and want to lose as much weight as possible in the least amount of time, another day without bread, potatoes, and pasta is exactly what you need!

As for the other kind of boredom, boredom with the need to be ever-vigilant, to watch what you eat, to adhere to strict rules and regulations, to curb all of your food impulses—that, too, is natural and inevitable after a few days on any diet.

Understanding the causes of your boredom is the first step in dealing with it. After that, it's a simple matter of not allowing boredom to get in the way of success. The suggestions that follow are designed to help you combat boredom on the Four-Day Wonder Diet. They should be equally useful in the future, if you decide to continue losing weight on a long-term reducing diet.

—Shake up your schedule, break with routine. Anything you do to relieve the sameness and regimentation of other parts of your life will lessen diet boredom, too. A spur-of-the-moment decision to lock up the office and take in a midafternoon movie, visit a museum or art gallery, or drive out to the beach or country can be extremely effective. So can the pleasure of spending unplanned intimate hours with your spouse or lover.

If you've been stuck in the house, get out. If you've

been keeping to yourself, seek company. If things have been deadly dull, anything you do to pick up the pace can work wonders. Conversely, if you've been madly busy, make an effort to decelerate and do something slow-paced and lazy. The important thing is to alter the circumstances and the tempo of your life, if only for a few hours.

—Treat yourself to something that will make you feel super-special. A present, even if it's only from you to you, is always a sure cure for boredom. Buy something great to wear, get a new hairdo, a manicure and pedicure, a facial, a massage. If you have to justify it to yourself, think of it as an advance reward for staying on your diet till the very end. (When tomorrow comes you won't *need* a reward; your final weight loss tally on the Four-Day Wonder Diet will be prize enough. Honestly!)

—Get busy! Make a list of all the chores you've been putting off, then roll up your sleeves and hit them with everything you've got. Although it's definitely not as much fun as taking time off from work or buying yourself a present, tackling the tasks that need doing is an excellent way to banish boredom. Answer your mail, pay bills, balance your checkbook. Reorganize your closets. Clean out the garage. Run out for some paint and brighten up the bedroom.

Almost any work that keeps your brain or your body fully occupied will also make time fly and take your mind off the dullness of dieting. Not to mention the fact that you will ultimately have something worthwhile to show for all that busy-ness.

DAY FOUR DINNER

For your final meal of the Four-Day Wonder Diet cycle, you will have as much broiled steak and lettuce and tomato salad (no dressing) as you like, plus a six-ounce glass of unsweetened pineapple juice.

It's only natural that you will be eager to get off the diet now and back to your normal eating habits—or, alternatively, to get started with a less restrictive, long-distance diet that will help you lose more weight over the coming weeks and months. You should remember, however, that even though this is your last dinner on the Four-Day Wonder Diet, the diet doesn't end when you finish the meal. There are a good twelve hours or so to go until final weigh-in tomorrow morning. Which means that you must follow the Four-Day Wonder Diet no-snack policy for the remainder of the evening.

This is no time to celebrate with food, so put all thoughts of late-night fridge-raiding out of your mind. You'll love yourself in the morning if you do.

END-OF-DIET SUMMING-UP

A valuable thing to do sometime this evening in the quiet hours before bedtime would be to reflect on your experiences with the Four-Day Wonder Diet while they're still fresh in your mind. Get out your diet journal and read over the notes and comments you made during the last four days. (If you didn't get everything down on paper, just try hard to remember.)

Ask yourself which times during the diet seemed easiest, and which more difficult, and see if you can figure out why. When did you feel most confident and full of energy, and when—if ever—were you ready to quit? Can you discern a pattern to these ups and downs? Do they seem to correspond in any way to the amount of food you ate? (Some people do feel better when they eat less.) Or to the amount of physical activity you engaged in? Or to conversations with family or friends? Is there a time pattern? (For example, did you consistently feel best in the mornings? Afternoons? Late evenings?)

The object, of course, is to try to achieve some insight into the factors that made losing weight easier for you at some times and less easy at others. This kind of insight will be helpful next time around on the Four-Day Wonder Diet. It will also increase your chances for success on other diets you may try in the future. It will help you understand which people, situations, and activities have a positive, confidence-building effect, and which to avoid, if at all possible. It will also alert you to the circumstances and times of day when you need to make an extra effort to stay on course.

Now, lights out and get some sleep. If you have any trouble dozing off, instead of counting sheep, try counting all the pounds you lost!

NINE

The 4-Day Wonder Diet: Day Five and After... How to Keep On Losing

YOU DID IT! You made the decision, followed the diet, and here it is, the day of reckoning. Now it's time to check final results. Get undressed, step on the scale, and enter the new pounds-lower weight in your diet journal. Take a few moments to admire the sleeker, tighter lines of your body. Then, while you're still undressed, get out the tape measure and see how you did in terms of shaping up through the bust and sculpting inches from your waist, hips, and thighs. Enter the new dimensions in your diet journal.

Of course you're elated with the pounds and inches you've lost. It's a safe bet that on looking back you'll wonder at the ease with which you were able to lose all those pounds on the Four-Day Wonder Diet. In fact, from today's vantage point it may seem *so* easy that you are tempted to start all over again immediately, and go back to Day One for a second round of the diet. Don't do it.

Allow at least four weeks to go by before you begin a second cycle of speedy weight loss on the Four-Day Wonder Diet.

HOW TO KEEP LOSING AFTER YOU'VE FINISHED THE 4-DAY WONDER DIET CYCLE

Suppose your goal is to take off fifteen, or twenty, or thirty pounds more than you have just lost on the Four-Day Wonder diet. Now is the ideal time to begin. You're flushed with success. Your motivation and self-confidence are at an all-time high. You've proved to yourself that you can deal with food cravings, stress, and boredom without losing control and going off your diet. And the total number of pounds you lost in the last four days will give you a head start in meeting your goal on any weight loss program you begin now. In short, you are perfectly positioned for success.

CHOOSING A DIET

The Four-Day Wonder diet put you on the fast track to rapid weight loss. Now, it's time for you to change over into the slow lane. As you know, many doctors with a special interest in weight control believe that the best way to take off a large number of pounds is to go on a diet that results in a slow and steady loss of between one and two pounds a week.

It is also important that the diet you choose to follow over a period of weeks or months be well balanced and include a variety of foods. Generally speaking, that means, on a per-day basis:

—Two or more servings of milk (skimmed or low-fat) or milk-based food such as cottage, pot or farmer cheese, or yogurt.

—At least two or three servings of vegetables. Ideally,

one should be a leafy green vegetable such as spinach or cabbage, and another should be a brightly colored vegetable, such as carrots or beets. On some diets, an occasional serving of pasta or starchy vegetable, such as corn or potatoes, is also allowed.

—Several servings of fruit, including one of citrus fruit. (A glass of orange or grapefruit juice counts as a fruit serving.) Often, fruit such as applesauce, sliced peaches, or strawberries, stands in for dessert after lunch or dinner. Also, fruit is often the midafternoon or evening snack of choice.

—Two or more servings of whole grain bread or cereal.

—One or more servings of meat, fish, poultry, or eggs. Meat is always roasted, baked, or broiled, never fried.

As you can see, there's plenty of good food to eat on a diet that includes all of the above.

On the no-no list for most good diets are junk food (such as potato chips and corn puffs), candy, butter, margarine, mayonnaise, salad oil and other fats, and often, but not always, pasta and starchy vegetables such as potatoes. No extravagant desserts are allowed, though some good diets do include an occasional small portion of ice cream or sherbet. And at least one—named after a major franchise diet organization—permits its own brand-name low-cal cake and cheesecake in certain circumstances.

By eliminating junk foods, restricting fats, starches, and sweets, and specifying smallish portions, doctors, nutritionists, and other experts are able to create diets that are healthy and at the same time low enough in calories that weight loss is the inevitable result of following them.

There's nothing mysterious about a good diet for long-term weight reduction. The best of them supply enough of a variety of foods to meet your body's minimum nutritional requirements, but fewer calories than it needs to maintain weight at its present level.

All of this may sound as though one well-planned, long-term weight loss diet is very much like the next. And in fact, there are more similarities between the best of the long-term diets than there are differences. You can count on losing weight on any one of them *if* you follow it correctly, and *if* the diet you choose supplies fewer calories than your body needs to maintain its present weight.

Most diets include information about the number of calories supplied daily. This is important information, as it will allow you to figure out for yourself whether a particular diet will in fact result in a steady two-pound-a-week weight loss for you.

HOW TO FIND YOUR OWN BEST CALORIE LEVEL FOR STEADY WEIGHT LOSS

Knowing the maximum number of calories you can eat and still lose approximately two pounds a week can enhance your chances of success on a diet. You can find out approximately what that number is by making a few super-simple calculations. But first, an explanation of basic diet dynamics.

Whether you're lean and lanky or a dumpling, your weight will stay where it is when you are in caloric balance and consume only as many calories each day as your body requires to sustain itself and function in all of the different activities you engage in. When your calorie intake equals your calorie output, your weight will remain at its present level. If your calorie intake is greater than your body's needs, the pounds will come creeping on. If you take in fewer calories than your body needs, pounds will gradually melt away.

To determine the approxmiate number of calories you can have each day and still lose about two pounds a week, you must know the number of calories required to maintain your present weight. The first step to doing this is to decide whether you are sedentary, somewhat active, moderately active, or quite active. (Be honest in your assessment; choose the most accurate description of you as you *are*, not the one that fits a fantasy image of yourself.)

Consider yourself "sedentary" if you're deskbound for most of each day and make little or no effort to engage in physical activities in your leisure hours. You're "active" if your job requires physical effort or you exercise vigorously several times a week. It's difficult to define precisely the two categories in between. However, if you think carefully about your *usual* daily routine, you should be able to place yourself correctly in one of these four slots.

If you are sedentary, multiply your present weight by 14.

If you are somewhat active, multiply your present weight by 15.

If you are moderately active, multiply your present weight by 16.

And if you are quite active, multiply your present weight by 17.

To illustrate, let's say your present weight is 150, and that you are only "somewhat" active. Multiply 150 by 15. The answer is 2,250, which means that if you consume close to 2,250 calories a day, your weight should remain steady at 150 pounds.

If you consume more than 2,250 calories a day, you will gain weight. How rapidly you will gain would depend, of course, on how many calories *more* than 2,250 per day you ate. For example, if you ate 100 calories more per day—the amount supplied by a large potato—you'd probably gain in the neighborhood of one fifth of a pound per week. Not much, but over a year, 100 extra calories a day would add up to about 10½ pounds!

Naturally, it works the other way, too. If every day you ate 100 calories less than your body requires, you would lose approximately 10½ pounds a year.

Once you know the approximate number of calories you need to maintain your weight at its present level, it's easy to figure out the number of calories per day that will result in a weight loss of about two pounds a week: Simply subtract 1,000.

(Why 1,000? Because there are 3,500 calories in a pound; 7,000 calories in two pounds, the amount you want to lose each week. Divide 7,000 calories by 7, the number of days in a week, and you get 1,000.)

To see how this works, let's again assume that your present weight is 150 pounds and that you are only somewhat active. To find the number of calories a day that will keep your weight more or less steady, multiply 150 by 15. The answer is 2,250 calories a day. To find the daily number of calories that should result in a weight loss of two pounds a week, subtract 1,000 from 2,250. The answer is 1,250.

Simplified, then, the formula for determining the number of calories that will result in an approximate two-pound-a-week weight loss for you goes like this:

> Multiply your present weight times 14 (if you are sedentary),
>> minus 1,000;
>
> Multiply your present weight times 15 (if you are somewhat active),
>> minus 1,000;
>
> Multiply your present weight times 16 (if you are moderately active),
>> minus 1,000;

Multiply your present weight times 17 (if you are quite active),
   minus 1,000.

ALL ABOUT "DIET SLOWDOWN"

Once you understand these simple weight loss dynamics, you will easily see why a diet supplying a specific number of calories might produce better, faster results for some people than for others. Imagine an active person weighing 170 pounds. That person would require 2,890 calories a day to maintain 170 pounds (170 times 17, the multiplier for active people) and should lose about two pounds a week on an allowance of 1,890 calories a day. That same person would lose weight faster than you would if you both went on the same 1,250-calorie-a-day diet (again assuming that you weigh 150 pounds and are only somewhat active).

These same weight loss dynamics help to explain the frustrating phenomenon of "diet slowdown" and why, over a period of weeks and months, it often takes longer and longer to lose each additional pound: As you lose pounds and weigh less, your body's caloric needs are reduced. Fewer calories are required to maintain your weight. And, all else being equal, the magic number of calories that will result in a two-pound-a-week weight loss becomes smaller.

To illustrate, let's again assume that you weigh 150 pounds and must limit yourself to 1,250 calories a day to lose two pounds a week. In five weeks you've lost ten pounds. But although you are following your diet as diligently as ever, your rate of loss is slowing.

You use the formula on page 86 and find that at your new weight of 140 pounds, you need to eat no more than 1,100 calories to continue losing weight at the rate of two pounds a week. The difference between 1,250 and 1,100 calories isn't that great, but it's enough to slow you down!

Adjusting your daily calorie intake downward as the pounds melt away is a little-mentioned but important technique in maintaining sure, steady weight loss over long periods.

HOW TO FINE-TUNE A DIET FOR STEADY, SURE WEIGHT LOSS

What if you *do* find that the diet you've been following has become "too big" for you, that it no longer produces steady, two-pound-a-week results? Ask your doctor about shaving a few calories off the diet you have been following (for each person there is a basic minimum number of calories necessary for good health and it would be unwise to consume fewer than that for an extended period.)

Assuming he or she gives you the go-ahead, there are a number of ways to adjust your caloric intake and output so that once again you will lose at a steady, sure rate. But first there is one thing you certainly should not do and that is to eliminate an entire food group. To do so would throw your diet out of balance and, possibly, lead to harmful deficiencies.

If you cut out the meat/poultry/fish/eggs group, for example, the overall calorie content of your diet would be lower, but you would also run the risk of creating a protein deficiency. (Some vegetarians *do* remain in good health despite a lack of food of animal origin, but they know how to combine other foods in ways that supply complete proteins. It is unlikely that your diet allows for such combinations, many of which consist of high-calorie legumes and grains.)

If you cut out the milk/cheese group, you'd be omitting important sources of calcium, a nutrient too important to good health to leave out of your diet for extended periods.

If you cut out fruits entirely, you'd be sacrificing major sources of vitamins and fiber. The same would be true if you eliminated vegetables.

To cut out breads and cereals would be to deprive yourself of good sources of fiber and B vitamins.

Far better and safer than eliminating any particular food group is to cut back a little on all of the foods on your diet. You can easily pare one hundred, two hundred, and even three hundred calories a day from a good reducing diet without upsetting its nutritional balance. Here are a few hints on how to do it.

Leave a Few Leftovers. One good way to cut back "a little" on everything is simply *not* to eat every morsel on your plate. Instead, leave a good-sized bite of each food. (Diet or no diet, leaving a small amount of food on your plate is an excellent habit to cultivate. If you don't go overboard on snacks and desserts, never have second helpings, and make it your policy not to polish off every scrap of first helpings, you may *never* have to diet again. Painless weight control.)

Decrease Portion Sizes. For some dieters, less steel-willed, it's easier to slightly decrease portion sizes at cooking or serving time. If you are on a diet that cals for exact weighing and measuring of food, give yourself an ounce less of meat, fish, or poultry at lunch and dinner, for example. Pour yourself six or seven ounces of skimmed milk instead of a full eight. Have half or three-quarters of a slice of bread instead of a whole slice. Use medium eggs instead of large. When you shop for peaches, apples, grapefruit, and other fruit, select the smallest specimens. As for vegetables, most of them are so low in calories that the number you'd save by serving vegetables in smaller amounts would be negligible. However, all other small adjustments are worth making. Taken together, the difference should be enough to start you losing weight again at a good, safe clip.

Get into Calorie Counting. If you are one of the not-so-rare dieters who actually enjoy poring over calorie-count books and you also get a kick out of toting up totals with a calculator, you might want to approach the whole business scientifically. You'll need a good, comprehensive calorie counter, one that lists not just "beef," for example, but all the different cuts of beef, from chuck to sirloin, along with the calorie count per ounce for each.

With one of these books to guide you, you'll quickly be able to identify the lowest-calorie foods in each group. Then make it a point to use those foods, whenever possible, to lower your daily calorie intake without substantially altering the nutritional balance of your diet.

A quick check through a good calorie book, for example, will tell you that four ounces of broiled club steak, trimmed of fat, has 277 calories; four ounces of broiled t-bone steak, trimmed of fat, has 253 calories; and four ounces of broiled sirloin steak, trimmed of fat, has 235 calories.

Or, if your diet specifies "a piece of fruit" for dessert or as a midafternoon snack, one of these books will steer you toward the lowest-calorie varieties. Cantaloupe, for example, at 60 calories for a half melon is a better choice than a cup of sweet cherries, at 83 calories.

If you're one of those who can't be bothered making precise calculations, this method of cutting back on calories obviously is not for you. But if you like the idea of keeping careful tabs on your calorie intake—and many do!—using a calorie counter to make fine-line distinctions between different types of foods can make a significant difference in your diet.

Be More Active. Finally, you can always boost your

calorie outgo instead of lowering your calorie intake. As you know, physical activity accelerates calorie burnoff. If you can find ways to "spend" an extra two hundred or so calories a day, you should be able to speed up your weight loss rate to the desired two pounds a week *without* cutting back on the food you eat. Furthermore, enough of the right kind of exercise will shape and firm problem areas and add to your overall sense of well-being. For more about exercise and how it can help, see Chapter Eleven.

POST–4-DAY-WONDER-DIET SUCCESS STRATEGIES

Though the food you ate on the Four-Day Wonder Diet was different from the meals you will be having on a regimen intended for long-term weight loss, many of the tricks and techniques that make dieting easier are the same. The Deep Breathing and Positive Picturing strategies for stress relief in Chapter Seven, for example, and the Bath Therapy mentioned in Chapter Six, can be used to enhance your chances for success on *any* diet. On the other hand, the suggestions below apply only when you are on a diet meant to be followed for longer periods, of a month or more.

Modify your expectations. This is especially important if you have just completed a round of the Four-Day Wonder Diet, resulting in speedy, significant weight loss. On the Four-Day Wonder Diet, you were geared up for immediate gratification—and that's what you got! Now you must make the adjustment to patient anticipation. Before, you were a sprinter. Now, try to think of yourself as a long-distance runner, with the heart and drive to pursue your goal for as long as it takes. Unless you make this shift in attitude, you will almost certainly be handicapped by a sense of frustration.

Paradoxically, a good way to avoid feeling frustrated is *not* to dwell on the long-range aspect of your diet, *not* to think about the number of weeks it will take to reach your target weight. Instead, focus on achieving success one day at a time. Forget about yesterday. Don't worry about tomorrow. Concentrate on getting through today. Every single day that you stay on your diet counts as a success and makes you a winner. As the days of your diet add up, so will your successes.

Say no to guilt feelings. If you do give in to temptation one day and go off your diet, *force* yourself not to get bogged down in feelings of guilt and worthlessness. Nobody's perfect. Everyone slips up occasionally. One chocolate ice cream cone or bag of chips needn't spell disaster to your diet *if* you limit the damage and don't allow yourself to go out of control. If you feel you must "pay" for a dietary indiscretion, "punish" yourself by eating less—or even nothing—at your next meal, or by doing enough walking, jogging, or calisthenics to burn off some of the extra calories.

Don't "over-weigh" yourself. Since you won't see fast, dramatic results on a long-term diet, stop weighing yourself each morning, as you did on the Four-Day Wonder Diet, when the daily weigh-in offered visual proof of rapid progress. Instead of keeping your motivation high, daily weigh-ins on a slower-working diet can have just the opposite effect. The best way to keep track of pounds lost on a long-term diet is to hop on the scale once a week only.

Give yourself frequent rewards. On the Four-Day Wonder Diet, rapid weight loss was its own reward. On a slower diet, you may need some additional help to keep your resolve from flagging. A good way to keep your morale high and your will strong is to give yourself something each time you lose a specific amount of weight. (Feedback from others is gratifying, but you can't always count on getting it when you need it most.)

Ideally, the reward you give yourself should be something meaningful, something you really want. (But not food, of course.) Your perfect reward might be a book you've been wanting to read, the latest issue of a favorite magazine, an evening out, an addition to a collection, hobby supplies, a plant. It's important that your reward be something you can give yourself *immediately* upon reaching the interim goal. If you have to wait too long for your treat, it will no longer be associated in your mind with the pounds you lost, and its morale-building effect will be lessened.

Surround yourself with reminders. The kind of reminder we're talking about here can be almost anything that forces you to confront your weight problem and reinforces your desire to solve it. An unflattering "before" picture, showing you at your bulgiest, can be a powerful reminder. Of course, it's useless unless you remember to look at it at critical moments. Many dieters have duplicate "before" pictures made—one to carry with them, and another to display in a prominent place, such as taped to the refrigerator door.

Tip: Have your refrigerator picture photocopied and enlarged to almost life-size so that it will be impossible to ignore!

The sight of your own body, stark naked, in a full-length mirror is another potent reminder.

Clothes that are now too tight to wear are excellent reminders, too. If you're at home when the need for a food fix hits, head for the bedroom and try on some of the old favorites you hope to be able to fit into again.

Tip: As the results of your diet become apparent, buy one or two flattering new things that enhance your slimmer shape. They'll give you a lift and at the same time they'll be all-day reminders, when you wear them, of the importance of sticking to your diet.

Have a diet buddy. Though talking about your diet to everyone and anyone can have negative effects (it will turn some people off, while others might try to dissuade you from losing weight), confiding in one special person can be helpful. That special person could be another dieter with whom you work out a mutual-aid relationship so that either will feel free to call the other in moments of need. You and your diet buddy can talk each other through the bad times, and cheer each other's successes. At best, a diet buddy can make losing weight easier and more fun. At the very least, you will both feel less isolated.

If you don't know anyone who is on a diet (unlikely, but possible), ask a good friend if you can call on him or her for support and encouragement. A warning: Parents and spouses often are not well-suited to the role of diet buddy. Their relationship to the dieter may be so complex and emotional that they are unable to give consistent and unqualified support. It is better to seek out someone who is loyal and true blue and who has your best interests at heart, but who is at the same time one or two steps removed from you emotionally.

HOW TO SET REALISTIC GOALS

How much weight do you want to lose? On the Four-Day Wonder Diet, the answer was easy: As much as possible, as quickly as possible. However, when you are dieting over the long haul, it is best to have a specific goal in mind. A goal will give you something to aim for and provide a valuable point of reference. With a goal, you will know when you've hit the halfway point, or reached the just-five-more-pounds-to-go mark.

You probably have some idea of what you want to weigh. (For many dieters, "ideal" weight is the weight at which they felt and looked their best at some time in the past.) But if you're not sure what your goal should be, a height-weight chart is a useful tool. No diet book would be complete without one of these charts, which indicate a range of ideal weights for women and men calculated on the basis of height and bone structure, or "frame size." This book is no exception.

Most people know within a fraction of an inch how tall they are, but if you want to re-check for accuracy, take off your shoes and stand tall against a wall. Your buttocks and the back of your head should be pressed firmly against the wall. Ask someone to mark your height by placing a book on your head (the book should be level and at a right angle to the wall) and marking the point where the book hits the wall. Now, with a yardstick, measure the distance from floor to mark.

How do you know if your frame is small, medium, or large? (Or, to put it another way, how can you tell whether you are small-boned, medium-boned, or large-boned?) A good way to find out is to measure your wrist at its widest point. (See that protruding bone on the pinky-finger side of your wrist? Measure around that bone.) If you are a woman, a measurement of less than six inches puts you in the small-frame category; a six- to six-and-one-half-inch wrist measurement tells you that your frame is medium; if you measure more than six-and-one-half inches, you have a large frame. A man with a wrist measurement of less than six inches has a small frame; six to seven inches indicates a medium frame; over seven inches and he has a large frame.

Results of the wristbone test for determining frame size are accurate in the great majority of cases, but not always. Some people's wrists simply are not in proportion to the rest of them. If your features are small, for example, and your hips, shoulders, and ribcage are narrow and yet, according to the figures above, your frame is large, chances are your wrist measurement doesn't reflect your bone structure. You are one of the exceptions. Take the discrepancy into consideration when you use the height-weight chart.

When all is said and done, height-weight charts are merely guidelines, valuable ones to be sure, but not necessarily the last word on what you ought to weigh. For example, a fashion model probably wouldn't be able to find much work if, at five feet eight inches, she weighed in at 125—a good weight for small-boned women of that height, according to the charts, but not thin enough for an ultra-chic image. In fact, many clothes-conscious women are convinced that they look their best when they weigh a few pounds less than what the charts indicate as ideal.

On the other hand, because muscle weighs more than fat, lean but heavily muscled athletic types are sometimes "overweight" according to the charts.

Take all the relevant factors into consideration when establishing your weight goal. Then use that goal as a target, something to shoot at. You might ultimately decide that you look and feel your best when you weigh a few pounds more or less than your goal. But you won't know that until you reach it. And you will!

MEN

| Height | | Small | Medium | Large |
Feet	Inches	Frame	Frame	Frame
5	2	128–134	131–141	138–150
5	3	130–136	133–143	140–153
5	4	132–138	135–145	142–156
5	5	134–140	137–148	144–160
5	6	136–142	139–151	146–164
5	7	138–145	142–154	149–168
5	8	140–148	145–157	152–172
5	9	142–151	148–160	155–176
5	10	144–154	151–163	158–180
5	11	146–157	154–166	161–184
6	0	149–160	157–170	164–188
6	1	152–164	160–174	168–192
6	2	155–168	164–178	172–197
6	3	158–172	167–182	176–202
6	4	162–176	171–187	181–207

WOMEN

| Height | | Small | Medium | Large |
Feet	Inches	Frame	Frame	Frame
4	10	102–111	109–121	118–131
4	11	103–113	111–123	120–134
5	0	104–115	113–126	122–137
5	1	106–118	115–129	125–140
5	2	108–121	118–132	128–143
5	3	111–124	121–135	131–147
5	4	114–127	124–138	134–151
5	5	117–130	127–141	137–155
5	6	120–133	130–144	140–159
5	7	123–136	133–147	143–163
5	8	126–139	136–150	146–167
5	9	129–142	139–153	149–170
5	10	132–145	142–156	152–173
5	11	135–148	145–159	155–176
6	0	138–151	148–162	158–179

Source of basic data: 1979 Build Study, Society of Actuaries and Associaton of Life Insurance Medical Directors of America, 1980.
Copyright 1983 Metropolitan Life Insurance Company

TEN

Day Five and After: How to Keep Your Weight Where You Want It

CHAPTER NINE FOCUSED on how to keep your losing streak going after you shed initial pounds on a round of Four-Day Wonder dieting. But what if the Four-Day Wonder Diet worked so well for you that in less than a week you lost *all* the weight you wanted to lose? Your primary aim now is to lock in those incredible Four-Day Wonder Diet results so that it will be a long, long time before you need to think of dieting again.

You know (perhaps from experience!) that if you throw all caution to the wind and begin to eat as though there'll be no tomorrow, your success will be short-lived. If you immediately and consistently consume more food than your body needs to maintain your new weight, the pounds will soon come creeping back on again. It's a dreary fact that most of us would prefer to ignore, but we do so at our peril.

HOW TO DETERMINE YOUR "MAGIC" CALORIE MAXIMUM

How do you know how much you can eat to keep your weight steady and your figure as sleek and shaped up as it is today? It's easy to find an approximate answer in terms of calories. All you have to do is make a single, simple calculation. The formula was given in Chapter Nine, but for your convenience, it's repeated here.

First, decide which description best applies to you:

Sedentary
Somewhat active
Moderately active
Active

To figure the maximum number of calories you can have each day without gaining weight:

Multiply your present weight times 14 if you are sedentary.

Multiply your present weight times 15 if you are somewhat active.

Multiply your present weight times 16 if you are moderately active.

Multiply your present weight times 17 if you are active.

For a closer look at how the formula works, let's assume that you now weigh 120 pounds and that you believe you belong in the "moderately active" category. Simply multiply 120 by 16. The answer is 1,920. Which means that to keep your weight steady at 120 pounds, you should consume in the neighborhood of 1,920 calories each day. If you consistently eat many more than 1,920 calories and do not at the same time become more active, you will gain weight. If you consistently eat significantly fewer than 1,920 calories, you will lose weight.

All of this calculating is a way of sketching in the broad

picture. You needn't plan your meals each day so that you end up with a perfect tally of 1,920 calories. In fact, to maintain your weight, you don't have to count calories at all, unless you want to. But you should spend some time looking through a good, comprehensive calorie book in order to familiarize yourself with the relative caloric values of different foods. Just an hour or so with such a book should tell you most of what you need to know to stay *approximately* within the calorie limits that will keep your weight down where you want it.

PACING YOUR EATING, MONITORING YOUR WEIGHT—THE KEYS TO DIET-FREE WEIGHT CONTROL

If you know the approximate number of calories you can have each day and still maintain your weight, and if you also have a general idea of which foods are very high in calories and which are low-cal, you'll be able to keep the pounds off by "pacing" your eating.

How is "paced" eating different from dieting? For one thing, it allows you unlimited choices. Love cannelloni? Have some! Got a yen for peanut butter cookies? Take a couple. With paced eating, you can enjoy all of your favorite foods without gaining weight as long as you don't overshoot by too much the magic number of calories that will keep your weight steady. When you do go over your limit, you can minimize the damage by cutting back on calories at the next meal, or the next day. You can even "bank" calories—save them up so that you'll have more to spend at a later date. For example, if dinner at a superb restaurant is on the agenda, you can eat less at breakfast and lunch, blow all of your savings in the evening, and not have to worry about gaining even a pound!

It's important to weigh yourself regularly in order to stay on track. Monitoring your weight once a day, or every other day, will alert you to a small problem before it has a chance to billow into a larger one.

If you enjoy the ritual of a daily weigh-in, keep in mind that daily weight fluctuations of a pound or so in either direction are the rule rather than the exception. These fluctuations are a result of water retention within the body, or reflect fluid intake, and are nothing to be concerned about. However, when the scale registers two or more pounds above your target weight, it's time to take action.

CAN'T-FAIL WEIGHT STABILIZING STRATEGIES

The Four-Day Wonder Diet offers a quick, sure cure for minor weight problems, but as you know, you must wait a month after finishing up one Four-Day Wonder Diet cycle before you begin another. In the meantime, the suggestions here will help you coax off the unwanted pound or so that stands between you and your ideal weight.

Take smaller portions of everything. (Leafy green and bright-colored vegetables are the exceptions. These you can load up on to your heart's content.) A good rule of thumb is to reduce portion sizes by about a third. If these smaller servings look depressingly skimpy on a dinner plate, use the golden-oldie dieter's trick of serving yourself on a salad plate!

Limit yourself to single servings. (Again, leafy green and bright-colored vegetables are exceptions.) Eat slowly, for maximum food satisfaction and to stretch out your meals. If you're still hungry by the time you reach the end of a meal, keep in mind that it takes a full twenty minutes for your stomach to register satiety, and that if you can only wait that long the craving for more food should disappear.

Choose low-cal but satisfying snacks. Fruit of any kind is always a good choice. (Instead of eating fruit "out of hand," American style, serve it to yourself in the European mode: on a plate, with a sharp knife for cutting it into bite-size pieces. Makes fruit seem more important, and thus more satisfying.)

Other good low-cal snack choices: a hard-boiled egg, seasoned with salt and pepper. A cup of bouillon. One or two kosher dill pickles with crisp melba toast. A half cup of low-fat cottage cheese. (Topped with a spoonful of dietetic jam or jelly, cottage cheese becomes a delicious "sundae.")

Make all sandwiches open face. Use a single slice of bread instead of two. Use less filling, and for greater eye appeal, garnish attractively with pimento, parsley, a lemon slice.

Have a meatless meal every other day. Steam up as much as you think you can eat of leafy green or bright-colored vegetables in any combination. Season with salt, pepper, herbs, spices, or lemon juice. If your meatless meal is lunch, try to have at least one good source of protein at dinner, and vice versa.

Avoid fats. Use nonstick utensils or one of the special noncaloric cooking sprays so that you won't need to add oil or butter to the pan when you scramble eggs, panbroil meats, and so forth. Trim all fat from meat and remove the skin from poultry before you eat it. In restaurants, order meat well done. (The longer cooking time allows more of the fat in meat to liquefy and run off.) At home, pat cooked meat with paper toweling to absorb excess fat before serving.

Eat your biggest meal of the day when you are most hungry. Have less (or even nothing, if your appetite is very small) at other times. There is evidence that food eaten late in the day, a few hours before bedtime, is more readily converted into fat than food eaten earlier. With this in mind, why not plan to make breakfast or lunch your biggest meal, at least once or twice a week, until your weight is back where you want it?

HOW TO MAKE EASY, PAINLESS SUBSTITUTIONS

Your efforts to keep pounds at bay and maintain the weight loss you achieved on the Four-Day Wonder Diet will be more successful if you learn how to substitute lower-calorie versions of the ordinary food you eat day in and day out. There are literally hundreds of easy, painless substitutions you can make—too many in fact to list in a book this size. There *is* space, however, to touch on a few of the most useful. (A quick read through a good calorie counter will turn up dozens and dozens of others.)

—Substitute plain (un-iced) angel food or sponge cake for layer or pound cake. Examples: A three-and-a-half ounce serving of pound cake has 475 calories; three-and-a-half ounces of chocolate layer cake has 369 calories; three-and-a-half ounces of sponge cake has 297 calories; and three-and-a-half ounces of angel food cake has only 269 calories!

—Substitute a plain (un-iced) cupcake for one with icing. Example: One white cupcake, iced, has 230 calories; one white cupcake plain has 115!

—Substitute ice milk or "no frills" yogurt (made without preserves) for ice cream. Examples: One cup of ice cream has 275 calories; one cup of ice milk has 199 calories; one cup of lemon- or coffee-flavored yogurt has 200 calories!

—Substitute fish or poultry for red meat, such as lamb, pork or beef. Examples: Four ounces of roast leg of lamb has 211 calories; four ounces of roast loin of pork has 411 calories; four ounces of beef rib roast has 273 calories. But, four ounces of broiled chicken has 160 calories. And four ounces of broiled flounder—prepared without butter—has 95 calories!

—Substitute plain vegetables for glazed or creamed. Four ounces of candied sweet potato has 190 calories; four ounces of plain boiled sweet potato has 108 calories. One cup of Harvard beets has 110 calories; one cup of plain beets has 65 calories.

—Substitute clear soup or consommé for creamed soup. Examples: One cup of cream of chicken soup has 180 calories; one cup of chicken consommé has 25 calories!

—Substitute a fruit or vegetable juice or grapefruit appetizer for pâté. Example: Two ounces of pâté has about 260 calories. A six-ounce glass of tomato juice has 38 calories; a half grapefruit has 60 calories.

—At breakfast, substitute ham for pork sausage. Examples: Three ounces of pork sausage has 400 calories; three ounces of boiled ham has 205 calories.

—At the movies, substitute pretzels for potato chips. Examples: Ten medium potato chips have 115 calories; ten small pretzel sticks have 35 calories.

Armed with the calorie-cutting lore in this chapter, and the determination to act on it, it should be possible for you to keep your weight on an even keel for months and months—without having to give up all of the foods you love best. Of course, exercise can also play an important role in getting your weight down where you want it and keeping it there. (For more about exercise, see Chapter Eleven.)

And then there is always the Four-Day Wonder Diet. Remember, you must allow a month to go by before starting a second round of the diet. After that, use it once again to chase away the pounds that plague you.

ELEVEN

Using Exercise to Maximize the 4-Day Wonder Diet Results

THE FOUR-DAY WONDER DIET will work for you regardless of how much, or how little, exercise you get. Eat the prescribed foods in the prescribed amounts, and your body will do all the rest. If you follow the diet faithfully, you'll lose up to ten pounds in less than a week, no matter what. You could lounge around in a pink negligee reading novels, and you'd *still* finish the four days pounds thinner.

BUT, if you combine the Four-Day Wonder Diet with a moderate increase in physical activity, the diet will pay off with even better results. It's impossible to predict or promise how much more weight you'll lose by being more active. The amount would vary according to your starting weight, as well as your age, size and musculature, and the kind and amount of exercise you get. But there's no disputing the fact that by increasing your level of physical activity you can maximize your weight loss on the Four-Day Wonder Diet.

Why is this so? As you know, increased physical activity will accelerate the body's rate of calorie burnoff. This increased calorie burnoff will take place whether you are on a diet or not. Think of it this way: If your body requires 2,000 calories a day in order to function and meet all the demands you place on it, and if the food you eat supplies you with exactly 2,000 calories a day, your weight will remain stable. You won't lose, and neither will you gain.

But if you continue to consume 2,000 calories' worth of food each day and at the same time spend an additional 100 calories a day by exercising, you will be creating a calorie deficit. In other words, though your calorie income remained at 2,000, your calorie outgo would be 2,100. All else being equal, if you continued to burn 100 calories more than you took in, you'd lose weight. Your weight loss would be slow. Since there are 3,500 calories in a pound, it would take you 35 days to lose a pound. But—again, all else being equal—lose it you would. And without cutting back on calories.

Keeping this vastly simplified explanation in mind, it's easy to see how increasing your calorie outgo—through exercise—can enhance the results you get when you reduce your calorie income by dieting.

But that's not the entire exercise story. Not only does your body burn calories at a faster rate *during* exercise, it continues to burn extra calories *afterward*, as well. Even if you do nothing but collapse into a chair and watch television after your workout, your body's calorie burnoff rate will remain elevated for as long as six hours. Of course, you won't burn off as many calories during the post-workout period as you did during the workout itself, but the increase can still be significant in melting away unwanted pounds.

There is some question among researchers as to how and why the body continues to burn calories at a greater rate after a period of exercise, but there's no disagreement that it does.

There's still more to the exercise story: Contrary to what many people have always taken as fact, exercise will not increase your appetite. It often has the opposite effect! Ordinary exercise—the kind that any normal person in good health is capable of doing—tends to suppress the desire for food for several hours after a workout.

Researchers are in greater agreement as to how exercise suppresses hunger than they are on the question of how calorie burnoff remains high after a workout. During increased activity, they say, the body produces more of a number of substances such as glucose, serotonin, noradrenaline and adrenaline, which depress the appetite. At the same time, less of the substances that promote hunger, such as cortisol and endorphins, are produced.

There is also evidence that regular, moderate exercise is *energizing*, that instead of tiring you out and slowing you down, it can perk you up and increase your capacity to enjoy a whole range of other activities that you might have felt too draggy to participate in in the past. In fact, many people who start a fitness program are amazed to discover that they not only do not need as much sleep as they did before, but also, paradoxically, when they do turn in for the evening they fall asleep more easily. (Of course *very* vigorous exercise, such as training for competitive sports and athletics events, or heavy, hard labor will indeed result in an energy drain and increase the need for sleep.)

If you're still not convinced, there's the fact that it's impossible to eat and exercise at the same time! Which means that by planning workouts for times when you're usually in the mood for food, you can keep yourself from temptation by, literally, walking, jogging, or swimming away from it!

HOW TO BEGIN? SLOWLY

The Four-Day Wonder Diet was created to get rid of pounds fast, with or without exercise. Once you've completed a four-day cycle, you can either start on a diet that will help you lose additional pounds at a slower rate, or eat to maintain your new, slimmer shape. As you've seen, stepping up your activity level can maximize the Four-Day Wonder Diet results, and make it even easier for you to keep on losing, or to stay at your ideal weight. But whatever your reason for exercising, it's important to key any new fitness program to your present physical condition.

Before you go out and buy new running shoes, join a gym, or check with the Y about pool schedules, talk to your doctor. Tell him or her what you have in mind and ask whether there is any reason why you should not begin a fitness program. Your physician may want you to come in for a checkup before giving a final okay.

Most exercise experts agree that people over the age of forty who haven't exercised during the previous year should plan to do no more than ten minutes of moderate exercise to start.

These same experts also warn that even ten minutes may be too much for some people, regardless of their age. If breathing becomes difficult, or you feel uncomfortable for *any* reason during exercise it's time to stop even if you've only been at it for a minute or two. In particular, be alert for signs such as pain in the upper body, abdomen, or arms, irregular heartbeat, a sudden speedup in heart rate, dizziness, feelings of faintness, or nausea. Any of these could mean that your heart is not functioning properly.

Even if you are under forty and in fairly good shape,

it's still important to go slowly during the first few weeks of a fitness program. You may discover that it's easy for you to do ten or fifteen minutes of your chosen activity without feeling tired. Great! But do stop as soon as your breathing begins to become difficult or your muscles start to feel heavy. To push yourself beyond that point would be to tax your heart unnecessarily and to court painfully sore muscles and even injury.

A good rule of thumb for anyone just starting an exercise program is to begin at a leisurely pace and without any particular goal—such as to walk or run or swim a certain distance or number of minutes—and to stop immediately when breathing becomes difficult or muscles begin to feel heavy. It may take a couple of sessions before you are able to better your initial distance or time, but within a matter of weeks, as your endurance and muscle strength improve, you'll notice a big difference.

The goal, according to many exercise physiologists, is to increase stamina and strength so that you are working out for half an hour a day, three days a week.

WHAT KIND OF EXERCISE FOR YOU?

Anything that gets you moving—striding, stretching, flexing, reaching, and so forth—will help you burn off additional calories and thus speed up weight loss on a diet. (Needless to say, it will also help you keep the pounds off when the goal is to maintain your present weight.) As mentioned earlier in this book, you can increase your total daily calorie expenditure enough to make a difference if you make the effort to do things the hard way: Do as many chores as possible "by hand" instead of relying on a plug-in appliance. Get off the elevator early and climb the last flight or two of stairs to your office.

Park your car a few blocks from the office and walk the rest of the way. And whenever you can, bike or walk instead of driving. Walk briskly instead of slowly. Stand when you could be sitting. None of these small changes are significant in themselves, but if you make enough of them, the payoff will be substantial.

However, the best kind of exercise for weight loss and fitness is the aerobic kind that involves continuous movement of the large muscles of the body (legs, especially, but also back and arm muscles).

Don't be fooled by that term "aerobic." To many people it implies simply a new kind of dance exercise. Aerobic dancing *is* a great way to shape up and achieve fitness, but it's far from the only aerobic exercise. Brisk walking is also aerobic. So are jogging, jumping rope, and jogging or running in place. So are bicycling and using a stationary bicycle, rowing and working out on a rowing machine. Swimming, too, is an excellent aerobic exercise.

Which of these would be best for you? First off, ask yourself which you'd enjoy most. (It makes no sense at all to plunge into an activity you loathe just because you think it will be good for you. In addition to the enjoyment factor, keep in mind when you make a decision that though all aerobic exercises are good calorie-burners and fitness builders, some will be better suited to your temperament, your schedule, and your skills than others.)

Aerobic dancing. You won't learn all the latest steps in an aerobic dance class. But you will be taken by a skilled instructor through a routine of vigorous movement, set to music. Classes will get you out of the house and introduce you to a group of like-minded others, which can be a big plus if you're a sociable type. In addition, signing up and paying for classes in advance should help keep you motivated. On the minus side is the cost of the classes, and the possibility, if you are self-conscious about your shape, that you will feel uncomfortable performing exercises in a form-fitting leotard.

Brisk Walking. This exercise requires no equipment other than comfortable clothing and shoes, doesn't cost a cent, and you can do it whenever you have a spare half hour or so. On the other hand, foul weather in summer and icy winter temperatures might weaken your resolve. (On some days you'll have to *force* yourself out the door.) Some people find that solitary walking is lonely, and it can be dangerous at certain times in certain neighborhoods. If you want or need company, see if you can get together at regular times with other walkers.

Jogging. Like walking, jogging requires no special equipment other than good shoes, doesn't cost anything, and can be fit into the most convenient time slot on your schedule. Needless to say, it's also very "in." However, the jolting movements involved in jogging are somewhat more stressful to bones and muscles than gentler walking motions. Also, you will occasionally be at the mercy of the weather. And solitary jogging can be just as lonesome or dangerous as solitary walking; a jogging group might be more fun and would certainly be safer.

Jumping rope and jogging in place. These can be done indoors when it's lousy outside, and outdoors when the weather is fine. Both are, like jogging, harder on bones and muscles than walking. (The exception is jogging in place on a mini-trampoline. This handy device "gives" with each step, cushioning foot-to-floor impact and thus greatly reducing stress on bones and muscles.) Doing anything "in place" is potentially a bore, since there's no change of scene. However, jumping or jogging in front of the television set can solve that problem.

Bicycling and exercising on a stationary bicycle. Both of these exercises require a substantial initial investment—unless, of course, you use a stationary bicycle at a gym or health club. (In that case, you will have to pay to use the facility.) However, either will give you a terrific all-over workout. Pluses and minuses: For outdoor cycling, there's the exhilaration of fresh air touring versus occasional inclement weather, traffic, and the odd overly playful dog. For indoor cycling, there's all-weather accessibility versus the tedium of working out "in place." (Again, if you can set up your stationary bicycle in front of the television you can watch as you pedal.)

Rowing and exercising on a rowing machine. Rowing is especially good for working the large muscles of the back, though legs, too, will benefit. Unless you live near a lake, rowing a boat will probably not be your primary choice for regular workouts. However, machine rowing indoors is a good, year-round activity. Television or conversation with other exercisers can alleviate boredom.

Swimming. This is another all-time great exercise, with the added plus that it is easier on the heart and less stressful to bones and muscles than many other activities. But first, of course, you must be able to swim. (Any stroke is fine; so is using a variety of strokes throughout your workout.) You must also have regular access to a pool. Though swimming isn't exactly a sociable activity, you probably will not be the only one in the water, unless you work out at odd hours, and soon after you start, you may find yourself with a host of new pool friends to keep you company.

The activities listed above certainly are not the only good calorie-burning and fitness-building exercises. However, many of the others, though effective and lots of fun, require special skills and are not as easy to do on a regular basis. ("Regular," in this case, meaning three times a week, thirty minutes a session.) Among these other excellent aerobic activities are roller-skating, ice-skating, cross-country skiing, fast ball sports such as racquetball, paddleball, squash and handball, and fast disco dancing. For extra weight loss benefits, why not try to do the ones you enjoy as often as possible, sandwiching them in one days when you do not engage in your primary activity?

Many people actually prefer to vary their exercise routine from session to session rather than concentrate on just one activity. Varying activities helps prevent boredom (an often-mentioned reason for quitting a fitness program), and since different exercises work different muscles in different ways, it assures good all-over toning, and allows muscles that are heavily used in one activity an opportunity to recoup as you participate in a different one. There is much to be said for a fitness program on which you jog one day, rest the next, swim on the third day, bicycle on the fourth, and so on.

If varying your exercise routine appeals to you, remember to ease slowly into each new activity. Once you have worked your way up to a full thirty minutes of one exercise, you will be in pretty good condition—but not necessarily in good enough condition to attempt a full thirty-minute session of a different exercise that uses different muscles. In other words, if you can easily swim thirty minutes without feeling fatigued or having breathing difficulties, don't assume that it will be equally easy for you to jog for thirty minutes. Work up to a thirty-minute jog slowly, just as you worked up slowly to thirty minutes of swimming. The same applies to any new exercise you want to add to your repertoire.

WARM UP, COOL DOWN

As every athlete knows, injuries—strains, sprains, tears, even breaks—are far more likely to occur when muscles have not been properly warmed up before vigorous activity. Many people who really ought to know better believe that warming and stretching are synonymous.

They're wrong. Stretching cold muscles is almost as risky as plunging directly into vigorous activity from a standstill. In fact, many athletes save stretching for *after* a workout.

A better way to warm up for an exercise session is to slide into your activity gradually and slowly. Slow walking—just ambling along—will warm you up properly for brisker walking. A slow, shuffling jog will get you ready for a faster pace. Slow, easy swimming will prepare you for more vigorous stroking. And so on.

How long should you spend on warming up? It depends on how far along you are in your fitness program. It may be that you will discover, when you first start out, that you can do no more than a minute or two of your chosen activity before you feel breathless and fatigued, no matter how slowly you pace yourself. In that case, you should perform at warmup speed for the duration of each session! Later on, as your endurance improves and your workout sessions lengthen to, say, fifteen minutes, you should spend five minutes or so at slow, warmup speed. When you're able to exercise for a full half hour, your warmups should last anywhere from five to ten minutes.

A cool-off period is important, too. It will help ease heart rate and circulation back to normal. It will also help prevent (or at least reduce) muscle soreness. Cool down as you warmed up, by continuing your activity at a slower pace for five minutes or so.

ANYONE FOR CALISTHENICS?

Calisthenics—those hup, two, three, four, toe-touching, body-twisting exercises that we all grunted and groaned through in high school physical education classes—are usually grouped separately from the aerobic activities we've been considering up to now. That is because calisthenics, unlike aerobics, are most often done in a series, with a short break or pause between the end of one exercise and the beginning of the next. In aerobics, movement is continuous, while in calisthenics, short bursts of movement are followed by short rests.

It is the continuous movement of aerobics, in fact, increasing the pulse rate and keeping it up high, that eventually results in the better heart and lung capacity that is a primary goal of fitness training.

Calisthenics are less valuable than aerobics when your goal is overall fitness. However, calisthenics *will* burn off extra calories and result in greater weight loss on the Four-Day Wonder Diet. (Remember, *any* exertion over and above what's normal and usual for you will increase your daily calorie expenditure.) Not only that, you can count on calisthenics to firm and tone specific areas of your body. A wisely chosen series of calisthenics, done properly over a period of time, will tone and tighten you up where you need it most.

To reiterate: A half hour of calisthenics won't contribute as much to heart health and all-around fitness as a half hour of aerobic activity. But calisthenics will accelerate calorie burnoff and help you lose more weight on the Four-Day Wonder Diet—and in the process make you smooth and sleek where once you were lumpy and loose.

Aerobics versus calisthenics? It's not an either/or proposition. They don't cancel each other out. They're complementary! Why not go for the benefits of both?

CALISTHENICS FOR TOP-TO-TOE TONING

Two Exercises to Shape and Firm Your Arms

1. GIANT ARM ARCS.

You'll need two weights for this one. But hold on, before you go out and buy weights, try this exercise with two books. They should be of approximately equal size and weight (between two-and-a-half and three-and-a-half pounds each) and easy to grasp.

    a. Stand erect, feet slightly apart, with your arms at your sides and a weight (or book) in each hand.

    b. Extend your arms to the sides at shoulder level. (If you are using books instead of weights, your thumbs should be on the *undersides* of the books.)

    c. Swing both arms forward and across your body in giant arcs. Keep your elbows straight and your arms at about shoulder level, but with your right arm slightly higher so that it passes over your left arm. Swing arms back to starting position. (This is one complete swing.) Now, swing them across your chest again, this time with your left arm slightly higher and crossing above your right.

    d. Repeat giant arcs, as above, alternating so that right arm crosses over left, then left arm crosses over right. Start with fifteen complete swings. Work up to forty.

2. ARM WEIGHT-WAIT.

You'll need weights or books for this one, too.

a. Lie on your back on the floor, with your arms extended over your head and a weight or book in each hand. Your hands should be resting on the floor.

b. Keeping your elbows straight, swing your arms slowly up around and down to your sides, to a point almost, but not quite, touching the floor.

c. Hold for a count of ten. Then swing your arms up and back behind your head.

d. Repeat ten times. Work up to twenty.

Two Waist-Shaping Tummy Flatteners

1. ROLL-UPS.

a. Lie on your back on the floor with your hands clasped under your head, your knees bent, and your toes hooked under a sofa or sturdy chair for ballast.

b. Slowly "roll" up, curling your neck, your shoulders, then your upper back up and off the floor until you are in a sitting position. (If you can't roll all the way up to sitting, roll up as far as possible. You will be able to roll up farther as your abdominal muscles—your tummy's natural "girdle"—gain strength.)

c. Slowly roll back down again, uncurling your back, shoulders and then your neck.

d. Repeat five times. Work up to fifteen.

2. BOUNCING BENDS.

a. Stand erect with your feet slightly apart, your right arm raised and curved over your head, your left arm hanging, relaxed, at your side.

b. Keeping your back straight, bend to your left at the waist and "bounce" five times, pressing your right arm slightly farther to the left with each downbeat.

c. Return to original position.

d. Repeat five times. Then raise your left arm and do five bouncing bends to the right. Work up to fifteen bouncing bends on each side.

Two hip-trimmers

1. FLEX KICKS.

a. Get down on the floor on your hands and knees.

b. Keeping your elbows straight, bring your left knee forward and up; at the same time lower your chin to your chest. The object: to touch your knee to your nose. (It doesn't matter if you can't actually make the two parts of your anatomy meet; just get them as close as possible.)

c. Straighten your left leg and extend it back and up as far as possible. At the same time, raise your chin from your chest and point it up toward the ceiling.

d. Repeat, this time bringing your right knee forward to touch your nose. Do ten flex kicks, alternating legs each time. Work up to thirty.

2. LEG ROLLS.

a. Lie on your back on the floor with your legs straight and together. Stretch your arms out to the sides. Your hands should be even with your shoulders and your palms should be on the floor.

b. Keeping your knees straight, slowly raise your legs until they form a right angle with the floor. Now, slowly lower your legs to the left. (Be sure to keep your right shoulder on the floor.) The object: To touch your left hand with your toes. (This is difficult; do the best you can.)

c. Slowly raise your legs, then slowly lower them to the right. (Keep that left shoulder on the floor.)

d. Start with eight leg rolls, alternating sides. Work up to twenty.

Two to Slim and Firm "Saddlebags" and Jelly Thighs

1. HALF SWIVELS.

a. Stand erect with your feet well apart, your arms open wide and your hands at shoulder level.

b. Shift your weight to your left foot. Swiveling from the hip, and without lifting your right foot from the floor, rotate it around and in to the left as far as possible. Still keeping your right foot on the floor, rotate it around and out to the right as far as possible. (The movement is something like grinding out a lit cigarette under the ball of your foot, only slower and more emphatic!)

c. Do fifteen complete swivels with your right foot, then shift your weight to your right foot and do fifteen complete swivels with your left foot. Work up to thirty swivels for each foot.

2. SCISSOR LIFTS.

a. Lie on the floor on your right side, with your right arm extended under your head. Bend your left arm at the elbow and place your left palm on the floor in front of you, for balance.

b. Keeping your knee straight, slowly raise your left leg as high as possible. Hold for a slow count of five. Then slowly lower it. Repeat five times.

c. Roll over onto your left side, reverse arm positions, then slowly raise your right leg as high as possible. Hold for a count of five, then lower it. Repeat five times.

d. Start with one set of five Scissor Lifts for each leg. Work up to three sets of five.

Two for Toned and Shapely Calves

1. KNEE FOLDS.

a. (This is another one to be done with weight or books.) Stand erect, feet together. Grasp a weight or book in each hand and place your hands at the back of your neck.

b. Rise up on your toes, then slowly "fold" at the knees into a deep knee bend. (Your heels should remain off the floor.)

c. Straighten your knees to bring yourself back into a standing position, then slowly lower your heels to the floor.

d. Repeat eight times. Work up to twenty.

2. SKIPS IN PLACE.

a. If you know how to skip, you also know how to do this exercise—only instead of moving forward, skip in one place! For those who do not know how to skip, try this: Run in place, but instead of shifting your weight immediately from one foot to the other, take a little hop first.

b. Skip in place until you begin to feel breathless, or your muscles begin to feel heavy.

MAKING THE MOST OF YOUR CALISTHENICS SESSIONS

Exercises are most effective when they're done rhythmically. As you work to discover the correct way to do the basic movements, you will also discover an inherent rhythm in those movements. Emphasize the rhythm—work with it, not against it.

Music will help you do exercises more rhythmically. It will also make calisthenics more fun. Any music that makes you feel like moving, snapping your fingers, tapping your toes, is the right music. And, yes, you *can* do slow exercises to fast music. The trick is to emphasize every fourth or even eighth beat instead of each and every downbeat.

Be just as cautious about beginning a program of calisthenics as you would be in starting an aerobics fitness program. Check with your doctor first. Be alert to danger signals, such as pain or discomfort in your upper body, arms, or abdomen, irregular or suddenly increased heart rate, feelings of dizziness or nausea, difficult breathing. If you have had back trouble in the past, take that fact into consideration, too.

If any exercise seems particularly difficult, don't strain to do it the suggested number of times. Rather, give yourself an A for effort, and do it only once or twice. Later, when you're stronger and more flexible, you will be able to work up to a greater number of repeats.

Keep in mind that it's the movement—the additional effort you expend—that will increase calorie burnoff and maximize your weight loss on the Four-Day Wonder Diet.

TWELVE

All of Your 4-Day Wonder Diet Questions Answered

IF YOU'VE READ this book straight through from the beginning, you now know everything you really *need* to know about the Four-Day Wonder Diet. You know how it works, why it works, what to eat and what not to eat ... as well as how to navigate your way through Days One to Four, and end up on Day Five pounds thinner, looking terrific, and feeling great about yourself and your success. Even so, don't skip this chapter. In reading the answers to questions asked by other Four-Day Wonder dieters, you will almost certainly discover information and tips that you can use to make your first round of the diet even easier and more gratifying.

Q. At the office, I almost always work through my lunch hours. Even at home I rarely eat lunch. However, I do enjoy a big breakfast and, frankly, grapefruit and black coffee just isn't enough. Is there any way to modify the Four-Day Wonder Diet to suit *me*?

A. On the Four-Day Wonder Diet, as on most other diets, the amount and kind of food you eat is more important than the time of day that you eat it. There are two good reasons why breakfast is the smallest meal on the Four-Day Wonder diet: First, a small breakfast, or even no breakfast, is in line with the preferences of many people. (Often, the no-breakfast people say they're in too big a rush to eat in the morning, though it's amazing how these same people manage to find the time to eat something on the run later in the day . . . a fact that leads inevitably to the conclusion that these people simply didn't feel like eating in the morning!) Second, a substantial breakfast often acts as an "appetizer," making the prospect of lunch even more welcome. Some dieters discover, to their amazement, that with a very small breakfast, such as the Four-Day Wonder Diet grapefruit and coffee, they feel less—not more—hungry in the middle of the day.

Apparently, it doesn't work that way for you. To go on a weight loss diet you must by definition accept the fact that you will have to make some changes . . . and even a few sacrifices. But if doing without a substantial breakfast makes you truly miserable, you might try moving your Four-Day Wonder Diet lunches into the breakfast time slot, and having the grapefruit at noon.

Q. Though I don't feel hungry after the Four-Day Wonder Diet dinners, I don't feel satisfied either. How can I control that awful urge to continue eating?

A. Don't linger at the table after dinner. When you've finished your meal, get up, head for the bathroom, and brush your teeth! This is an old standby trick used successfully by many ex-smokers. Just as it seems to lessen the desire to light up at the end of a meal, it also diminishes the desire for more food. Brushing your teeth freshens your mouth, leaves a slightly sweet taste (almost like dessert!) and puts a period at the end of your meal.

Another idea: One dieter reports that she finds it helpful to get up and wash the dishes immediately after dinner . . . even though the job officially belongs to her daughter.

Clearing the table, stacking, then washing and drying all the dinner things keeps her busy and her mind off food. By the time she's finished with the job, her stomach has begun to send out satiety signals and the strong desire to eat disappears. (Remember, it takes about twenty minutes after a meal for the stomach to register fullness.)

Q. Should I take a vitamin and mineral supplement while I am on the Four-Day Wonder Diet?

A. If you've been taking such a supplement all along, there is certainly no reason to stop while you're on the diet. As to whether you should start taking a supplement when you begin the diet, that's entirely up to you.

It has been emphasized several times in these pages that no matter how thrilled you are with your success on the Four-Day Wonder Diet, on the fifth day you must return to normal eating—or start a well-balanced reducing diet that includes a wide variety of food. That's because the Four-Day Wonder Diet does not supply you with enough of all the nutrients your body needs over the long haul. However, there's nothing at all to worry about in the short run.

To sum up. If it will somehow make you feel better to take a supplement, go ahead. But it's not necessary.

Q. Over the years I've developed a dislike of red meat. I'd love to try the Four-Day Wonder Diet, but the idea of eating all that beef turns me off. Couldn't I make some substitution?

A. Most people enjoy red meat. In fact, it's the steak, hamburger, and lamb chop that make the Four-Day Wonder Diet so appealing and the meals so satisfying to most dieters. But since those are the very foods that are preventing you from reaping the incredible fast weight loss benefits of the diet, yes, you can substitute more poultry (but not duck; it's too fatty) and some seafood for the red meat. Chicken, of course, is already an important part of the diet; seafood, which is also animal protein, has a high fat-burning capacity, like beef and lamb.

Among the best seafood choices are shrimp, scallops, lobster, clams, tuna (packed in water, not oil), and non-fatty fish, such as sole and flounder, and halibut. Mackerel, sardines, anchovies, herring, and salmon are less desirable.

It's important to steam or broil fish and shellfish with no butter or margarine. Breading and frying are, of course, no-nos.

If you choose the seafood alternative, be sure to be guided by the Four-Day Wonder Diet specifications with regard to quantity and amount. For example, on Day One, when you may have all the steak you want, you can, if you're not eating red meat, fill up on poultry or seafood. But on Day Two, when a single lamb chop is specified at lunchtime, you must limit yourself to a single four-ounce serving of poultry, fish, or shellfish.

Q. My biggest problem on a diet is that I can't keep my mind off food. I become so obsessed with it that it's difficult for me to concentrate on my work. (As soon as I finish lunch, I begin counting the hours and minutes until dinner.) At home, I'm drawn to the refrigerator like a moth to a flame. Is there a "cure" for this obsession?

A. Yours is a very common problem, and it's also a real toughie—which is why there has been so much emphasis in this book on activities that will keep you busy and occupied with matters other than eating. In essence, staying occupied is the cure.

It has worked for others and *it will work for you* if you will only give it a chance. A little soul-searching may be necessary here. It's important to understand yourself well enough to know what activities you really *can* lose yourself in. Everyone has a few such activities. They're not always fun, but they *are* absorbing.

Some people become totally absorbed, for example, in knitting or crocheting. (If you know how to do either, why not start a sweater or jacket when you start your diet? Pull out your handiwork and go to it whenever you have a free moment. By the time you're finished, you'll be pounds thinner and have something smashing to wear with your smashing new figure!) Gardening is another possibility. Or perhaps you become totally engrossed in acrostics, crossword puzzles, and other word games. Reading can be good if you're lucky enough to find a book you can't bear to put down.

The important thing is to take this suggestion seriously. We've all run across solutions to problems that seemed to make sense, but there's no way these solutions can work for us if we don't actually apply them.

P.S. If food wins out consistently over work for your attention at the office, maybe it's because you're not busy enough. Why not volunteer to take on an extra project and score points with the boss even as the pounds melt away?

Q. Special low-cal foods such as diet salad dressing and diet gelatin dessert would add variety and taste appeal but very few calories to the Four-Day Wonder Diet. Why aren't they allowed?

A. It's true that the special foods you mention are so low in calories that they would not add significantly to daily totals on the Four-Day Wonder Diet. But calories are not at issue here. Neither is the fact that these foods make meals more appealing and eating more fun. That's the reason why they're allowed on most other diets. And, paradoxically, that may also be the reason why those other diets are so difficult to follow.

On the Four-Day Wonder Diet the joys of food and the pleasures of eating are purposely de-emphasized. Think about it a moment and this Spartan approach will begin to make sense. After all, dieting is hard enough without dressing up your meals with extras—even low-cal extras—to make them even more enticing. The Four-Day

Wonder Diet no-frills policy may seem arbitrary at first, but the rationale is sound. More important, it's effective!

Q. I hate vegetables. Can't I just skip all the beans and salad greens on the Four-Day Wonder Diet and fill up on more meat instead?

A. No. Vegetables are an important part of Four-Day Wonder Diet eating. They add bulk to the diet and thus help prevent constipation, which can be a problem in all-protein diets. Not only that, the vegetables help satisfy the dieter's need to chew and swallow at a very low cost in calories, and they take up space in your stomach, contributing to feelings of fullness after a meal. Not to mention the fact that they're a good source of vitamins not supplied by the meat on the diet.

If you absolutely cannot tolerate one or more of the vegetables on the Four-Day Wonder Diet—either because you're allergic to them or because the taste makes you sick—you may have other vegetables in their place. Make your selections from among the substitutions listed in Chapter Three.

But eat vegetables you must! Otherwise you'll miss out on important Four-Day Wonder Diet advantages...in fact, you'll miss out on the diet. No vegetables, no Four-Day Wonder Diet.

Q. Dieting was so much easier before I got married. In those days I never brought into the house any food I wasn't supposed to eat. My refrigerator and the kitchen cabinet looked like Mother Hubbard's. With my husband around, there's food everywhere. Are there any tricks to dieting in the midst of plenty?

A. The sight of food in the fridge and on shelves— and on someone else's plate—certainly can make dieting more difficult. What you need to do is minimize your contact with food. If you can enlist your husband's co-operation, so much the better.

Stow leftovers in opaque containers or wrap them in

foil so that when you open the refrigerator you'll see "packaging," not the food itself.

Place the foods for which you have a special weakness way back in the darkest, most inaccessible corner of the highest shelves of your kitchen cabinets. (Naturally, these goodies will be equally inaccessible to your husband. See why cooperation and understanding are important?)

See if you can get him to do all the food shopping for the duration of your diet. If he also puts the groceries away you won't even *know* what calorific delights might be lurking at the backs of your cabinets.

Work out a deal whereby *he* clears the table after meals (in addition to wrapping and stashing leftovers, and scraping bits of food too small to save into the garbage), and *you* wash, dry, and put away the dishes. This will minimize your contact with tempting tidbits that you might otherwise feel the urge to pick at.

Q. I've heard a lot of criticism of the popular high-protein diets. Since the Four-Day Wonder Diet is a high-protein diet, don't the same criticisms apply to it as well?

A. The most highly criticized of the diets you refer to are the ones on which the dieter is instructed to eat virtually nothing but protein. In fact, high-protein is a misnomer when applied to these diets. It would almost be more accurate to call them "all-protein, all fat," since the dieter is encouraged to eat as much as desired of meat and fish, poultry and eggs, cheese, and on some, even bacon and mayonnaise, but very little or no vegetables or fruits or grains are permitted.

There is an obvious and very important difference between these all-protein, all-fat diets and the Four-Day Wonder Diet: Plenty of vegetables and some fruits are not only allowed on the Four-Day Wonder Diet, they're absolute musts. And because they are, the major criticisms aimed at the all-protein, all-fat diets don't apply.

Those criticisms have less to do with the effectiveness

of all-protein, all-fat diets than with their possible health consequences over extended periods. By their very nature, these diets are high in cholesterol and deficient in bulk and many vitamins. Eating only protein foods can result in the accumulation in the body of ketones, which can lead to nausea and fatigue. Excessive protein can also be dangerous to those whose kidneys do not function normally.

The Four-Day Wonder Diet *is* high in protein, but it is loaded with vegetables and fruit as well, and this fact places it in a category far removed from that of the all-protein, all-fat diets. So does the four-day time limit. In fact, the Four-Day Wonder Diet is in a class all by itself!

Q. Exercise is encouraged as a way to speed up weight loss on the Four-Day Wonder Diet. Would massage also be helpful?

A. Only in an indirect way. To lie there passively, without moving a muscle, while someone gently kneads and pummels your body can be highly pleasurable. But it won't help you burn off extra calories for the very simple reason that you are not doing any of the work. (On the contrary, the person who benefits from increased calorie burnoff during massage is the masseuse!)

However, there is certainly something to be said for massage if it makes you feel calmer and more relaxed, especially if you're the kind of person who turns to food in response to stress. Massage, by easing tension, might indeed also help you control the impulse to reach for something to eat . . . at least temporarily.

And massage, because it has a way of making you feel pampered and cared for, can also make you feel less deprived when you're on a diet. When the desire to indulge in something utterly delicious and sensual takes hold, a no-calorie massage could be every bit as satisfying as a zillion-calorie hot fudge sundae!

Q. What if I slip up on the Four-Day Wonder Diet,

and eat something that isn't on the diet? Would it cancel out the results of the other three days?

A. A lot depends on what you mean by "slipping up." A single cookie or a few potato chips on one day shouldn't undo completely all the good you accomplished on the other three. (After all, when you are trying to get your weight down, three days of dieting are certainly better than no days of dieting! Even *one* day on the Four-Day Wonder Diet puts you ahead in the fat-fighting game!) But any slip-up *will* prevent you from deriving maximum benefits over a four-day period.

The important thing, if you do slip up, is not to be too hard on yourself, not to let a single small lapse fill you with so much self-loathing that you despair of ever being able to stick to a diet and go off into a wild eating binge. If you feel you need to get even with yourself for falling off your diet, a better way to do it is to force yourself to get right back on again!

Q. My mother always uses food to express her love, even when I'm on a diet. When I go to visit, she cooks elaborate meals and then acts hurt when I don't eat. How can I handle her when I start on the Four-Day Wonder Diet?

A. Diet saboteurs—and your mother seems to be one of them—come in all shapes and sizes, and act as they do out of a variety of motivations. Parents, especially mothers, tend to show love and concern for their children by feeding them. A rejection of food is sometimes misinterpreted as a rejection of their love.

Couldn't you simply explain to your mother that it is very important to you to lose a few pounds, and that what you would *really* appreciate when you visit her is a meal that doesn't violate your diet? By letting her know specifically what food you *can* have, you'll be enlisting her support—in effect, including her instead of rejecting her. Chances are she'll be thrilled to cooperate. And if that doesn't work, perhaps you can simply avoid seeing her for the few days you'll be on the Four-Day Wonder Diet. If you need to stay in touch, you can always phone her.

Some diet saboteurs are motivated by insecurity or jealousy. For example, a desire on the part of someone they care about to become more attractive can make friends, lovers, even spouses, feel threatened. The result can be subtle attempts to undermine the diet. Others, spoilsports at heart, simply cannot tolerate the idea that the dieter has mustered the courage and fortitude to do something that they themselves cannot do: make changes for the better.

Whatever their motives—and very often, those motives are buried deep down beneath the surface of the consciousness—the diet saboteurs can undermine your efforts in a number of ways: by urging you to eat things that you shouldn't ("One little bite won't hurt"); by attempting to convince you that you don't need to lose weight ("You look great just as you are!"); by criticizing your diet ("It's too strict," or, "How can you lose weight if you eat all that meat?"). Often, such comments are delivered with all the good will in the world.

Rather than go on the defensive and argue with saboteurs about how and why you want to lose weight, try a firm, good-humored restatement of your intention to take off pounds. If you can then find a way to divert the conversation *away* from dieting, so much the better.

Better still is simply to keep quiet about your diet. If you need excuses for not eating as usual, you can always say you're not hungry. Or that you're in the mood for meat (on the Four-Day Wonder Diet steak, chop, and hamburger days). Or that you have this incredible craving for vegetables (on Day Two, when dinner is vegetarian).

The Four-Day Wonder Diet is over and done with so quickly, it shouldn't be too difficult to carry off this ploy.

Afterward, you can reveal the secret of your suddenly slimmer shape.

Q. As I get older, it takes longer and longer for me to lose a few pounds. The Four-Day Wonder Diet promises a weight loss of up to ten pounds in less than a week, but I'm skeptical. Can I really expect to lose that much on the diet?

A. Metabolism—the rate at which calories are burned—typically slows over the years. This is partly a function of aging, but a decrease in physical activity no doubt has something to do with it as well. After all, most people have less opportunity and inclination to exercise as they progress through middle age.

It's impossible to predict, let alone guarantee, how much an individual will lose on any particular diet, including, of course, the Four-Day Wonder Diet. Age isn't the only factor that determines the rate at which you, or anyone, will lose: Height, body build, present weight, and the amount of exercise you get all enter into the equation, too. But it is safe to predict that *you will lose as many pounds as you are capable of losing*—given all the variables—if you follow the Four-Day Wonder Diet exactly!

Q. My teenage daughter is eager to lose five pounds before school starts next week. Should I suggest that she go on the Four-Day Wonder Diet?

A. The person best qualified to answer this question is your daughter's physician. The answer you get will most certainly depend on your daughter's age, her degree of physical maturity, and the state of her health, among other things.

Many doctors—perhaps most—do not encourage their young patients to lose weight by dieting except in cases of extreme obesity. Rather, they suggest cutting back on snacks, substituting fruits and crunchy raw vegetables for junk food, and eliminating second helpings of foods such as mashed potatoes with gravy, french fries and other high-calorie teenage favorites.

Teenagers, especially figure-conscious girls, are notoriously bad eaters, with many of them alternately stuffing themselves and fasting—literally! To some parents, a modified version of the Four-Day Wonder Diet (minus the restrictions on snacks and milk and with the addition of a serving or two of bread and cereal) would seem to be a vast improvement over their teenager's "normal" eating habits. However, the decision really should be left to a doctor.

Q. I've been on a diet for three weeks now and have only a five-pound loss to show for it. The instructions for my diet say that it is important not to deviate from the food plan in any way; otherwise the diet won't work. But losing so slowly is discouraging. Would it help if I went on the Four-Day Wonder Diet?

A. Most probably. Sounds as though your present diet is one of those designed for slow, steady weight loss over a period of weeks and months. And slow it is! Switching over to the Four-Day Wonder Diet should help you lose several pounds in a hurry, and in the process boost your morale and steel your will to continue losing weight on your present diet.

Remember, you must go back to normal eating or resume your present reducing diet when you've finished with the Four-Day Wonder Diet. (Granted, you may be so delighted with the results you'll want to stay on it for a few more days, but don't.) However, if you are still dieting a month from now, and want another quick weight loss pickup, you can always go back for a second round of the Four-Day Wonder Diet to speed you on your way!

A SELECTED LIST OF HEALTH AND DIET TITLES AVAILABLE FROM BANTAM BOOKS

☐ 20729 6	**Dr. Atkins' Diet Revolution**	*Robert C. Atkins, M.D.*	£1.75
☐ 23546 X	**Aerobics**	*Kenneth Cooper M.D.*	£1.95
☐ 17191 7	**The 4 Day Diet**	*Margaret Danbrot*	£1.50
☐ 34067 0	**Quit Smoking in 30 Days**		
		Gary Holland and Herman Weiss M.D.	£1.50
☐ 23827 2	**The Herb Book**	*Edited by John Lust*	£2.95
☐ 17157 7	**Pritikin Promise**	*Nathan Pritikin*	£2.95
☐ 23148 0	**Getting Well Again**	*Carl & Stephanie Simonton*	£2.50
☐ 17203 4	**The Complete Scarsdale Medical Diet**		
		Herman Tarnower & Samm Sinclair Baker	£2.50

All these books are available at your bookshop or newsagent, or can be ordered direct from the publisher. Just tick the titles you want and fill in the form below.